MED'TOONS

Stephen Goldberg, M.D.

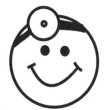

MedMaster, Inc., Miami
http://www.medmaster.net

10/31/99

Enjoy the book — Have many
Laughs — Happy Birthay Miss Betty,

With love always

Ray

Made in the United States of America

Published by
MedMaster, Inc.
P.O. Box 640028
Miami FL 33164

ISBN #0-940780-40-2

TO HEALTH CARE PROVIDERS AND PATIENTS
ALIKE, TO PROVIDE A BRIEF RESPITE FROM
THE STRESSES OF ILLNESS

THE AUTHOR: Dr. Stephen Goldberg has a uniquely combined career as a neuroanatomist and family physician. A graduate of the Albert Einstein College of Medicine, he subsequently trained in Neurology, Ophthalmology, and Family Medicine, with Board Certification in the latter two fields. Since 1975, he has instructed students at the University of Miami School of Medicine as Associate Professor in the Department of Cell Biology and Anatomy and Department of Family Medicine.

OTHER BOOKS BY THE AUTHOR:

Clinical Neuroanatomy Made Ridiculously Simple
Clinical Anatomy Made Ridiculously Simple
Clinical Biochemistry Made Ridiculously Simple
Clinical Physiology Made Ridiculously Simple
Ophthalmology Made Ridiculously Simple
The Four-Minute Neurologic Exam
Goldberg's Brain Model
Jonah: The Anatomy of the Soul
The Jonah Principle: The Basis for Human and Machine
        Consciousness
Consciousness, Information, and Meaning: The Origin of
        the Mind

CONTENTS

PREFACE

Humor is a form of therapy. Hopefully, this little noneducational book of medical cartoons will reduce, for a brief window of time, some of the tensions of the medical care system that are experienced by physicians, nurses and other health care professionals, students and patients.

The cartoon ideas, which may be characterized essentially as nonsense, were designed by the author, with no particular pattern in mind, except those thoughts that sprang to mind in daily walks. I prepared most of the cartoons using computer clip art along with Adobe Illustrator and Adobe Photoshop. A number of hand-drawn cartoons were drawn by Steve Goldberg (no relation), a brilliant former student of mine at the University of Miami School of Medicine who could have pursued an excellent career in illustration, but for some reason elected to enter a pediatric cardiac surgery residency. I thank Miguel Luciano for drawing the Cinderella cartoon and Conrad Barski for drawing the veterinarian chaos and menage a trois cartoons. I thank my wife Harriet, daughter Rebecca, Adam and Shaani Splaver, and my friends, the well-know humorist Larry Tuchinsky, and Marty Hoffman (who encouraged me greatly by actually laughing at some of the cartoons) for their pertinent comments, which led to the fortunate elimination or modification of a number of the illustrations.

Stephen Goldberg

ALTERNATIVE MEDICINE

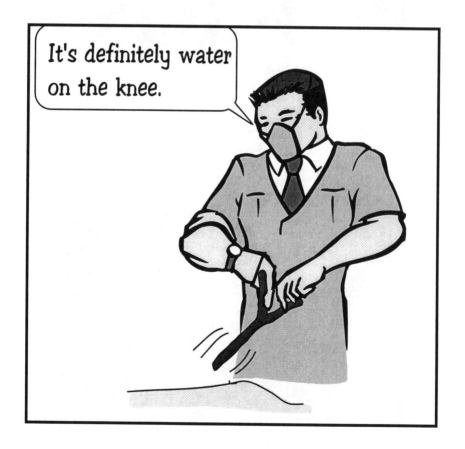

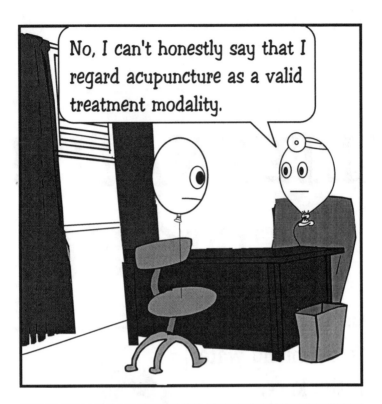

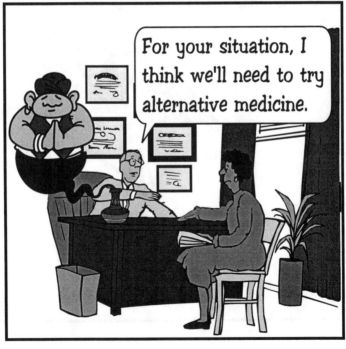

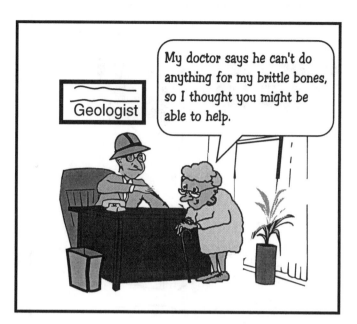

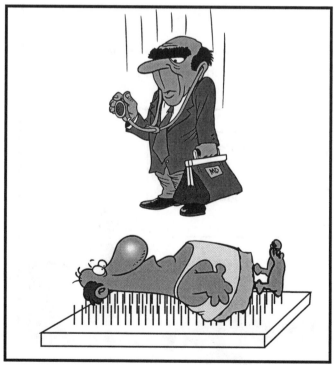

Instant acupuncture.

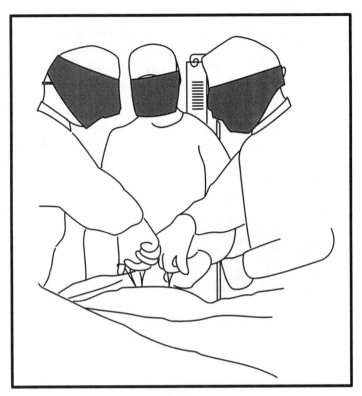

Psychic Surgery

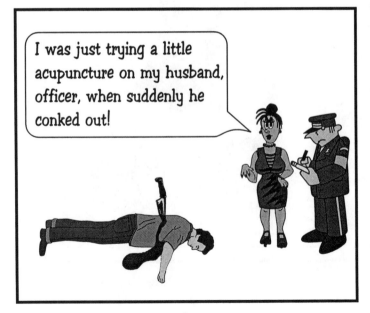

CARDIO-

PULMONARY

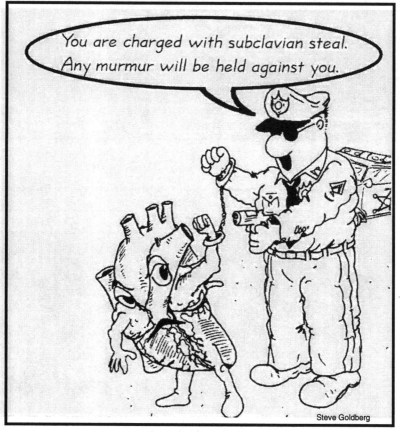

Cardiac arrest

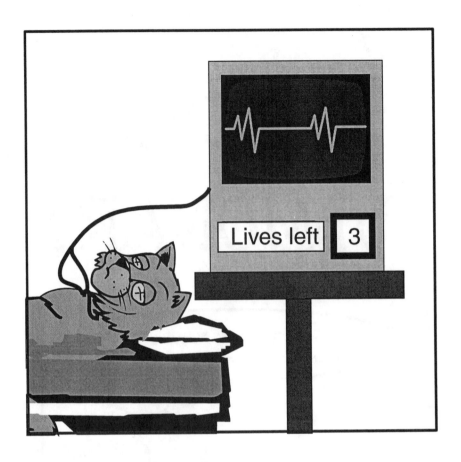

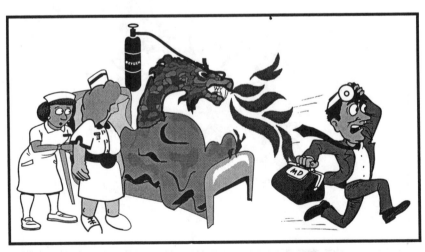

Perhaps oxygen wasn't such a good idea.

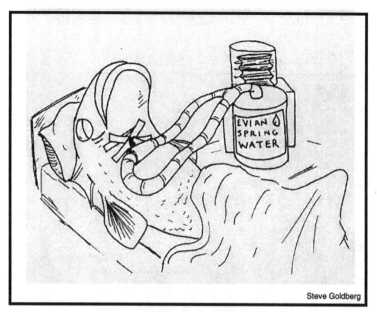

Fish respirators

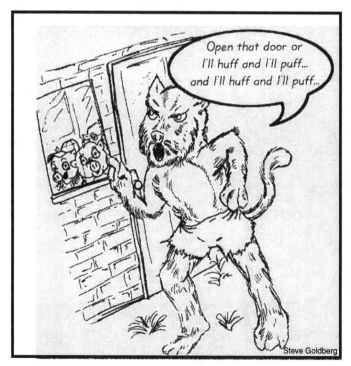

Emphysema in wolves

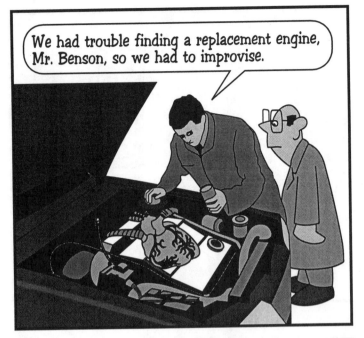

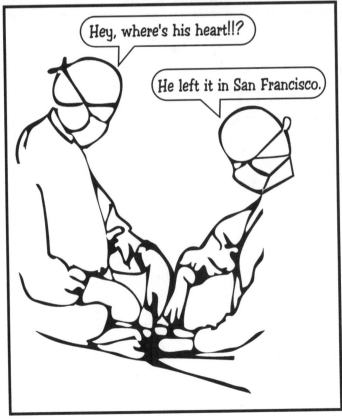

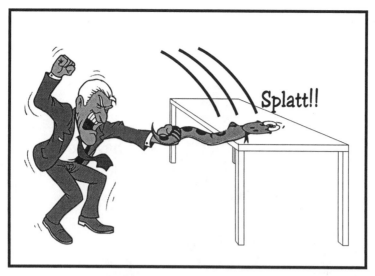

Heimlich maneuver in snakes.

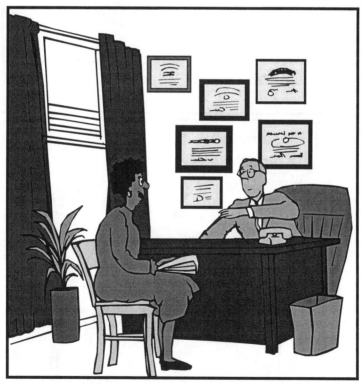

"I'm so happy with my new pacemaker, doctor. I can hardly wait to get back to my job as a microwave oven tester.

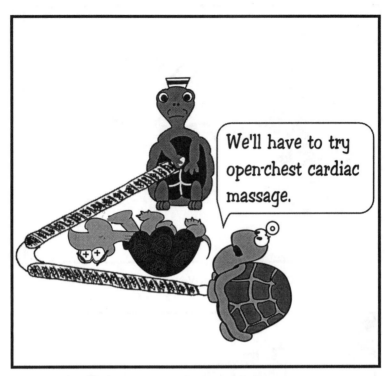

Heroic measures during cardiac arrest.

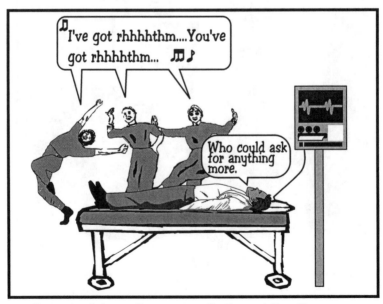

Successful cardiac resuscitation at the George Gershwin Memorial Hospital.

DEATH
&
DYING

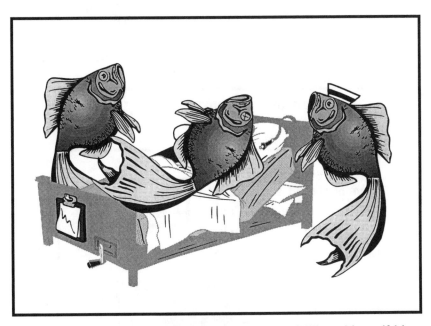

"Sorry about your husband's death, Mrs. Miller. Now, if it's O.K. with you, we have to move him over to the toilet."

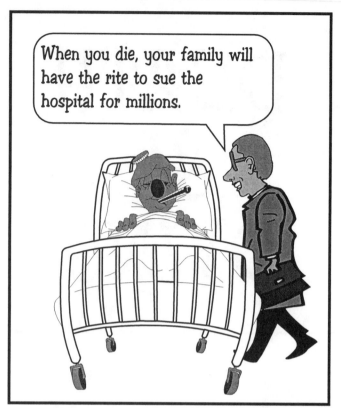

When lawyers administer "last rites."

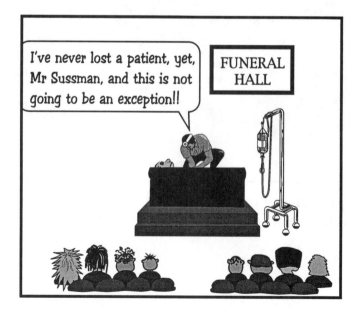

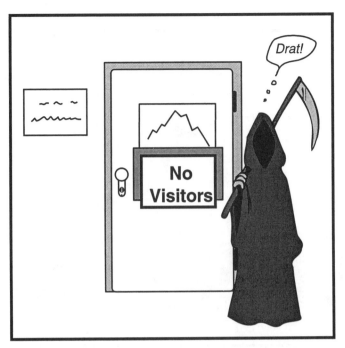

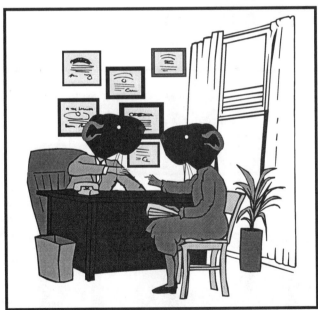

"Well, Mrs. Hamster, we can do the cardiopulmonary transplant on your husband, or, at less expense, we can just discard him and buy another one."

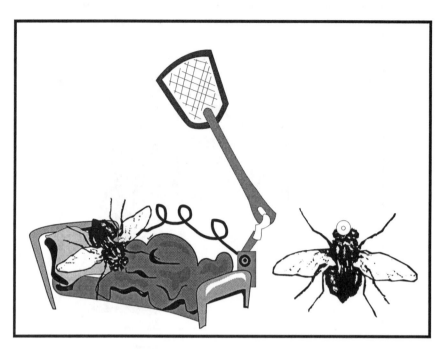

Dr Flyvorkian strikes again

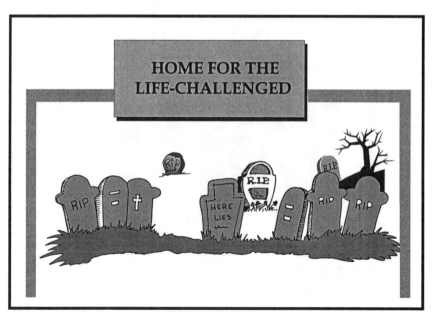

Political correctness comes to death

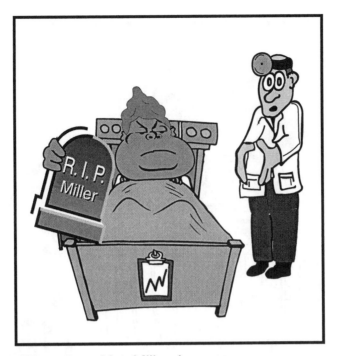

"Now, now, Mrs. Miller, I assure you your pessimism about your operation tomorrow is greatly exaggerated."

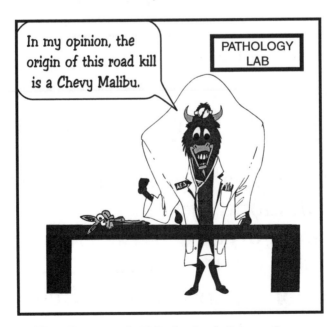

The fine art of pathological diagnosis.

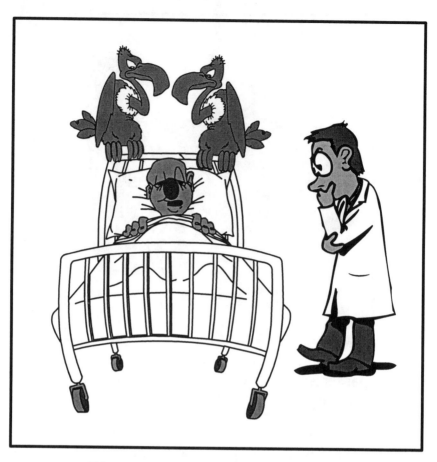

"How am I doing today, doctor?"

ORGAN DONOR CARD

In case of death please donate my:
☐ Hammond organ
☒ Kawai organ
☐ Other organ _____
to St. John's Episcopal church

DERMATOLOGY

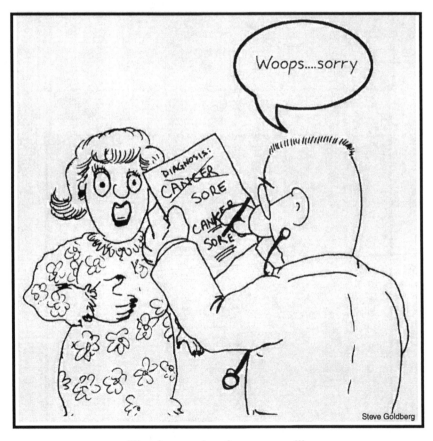

The hazards of poor spelling

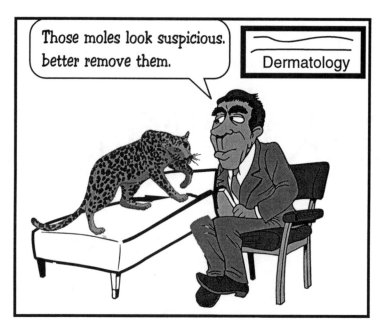

Fraud in dermatology.

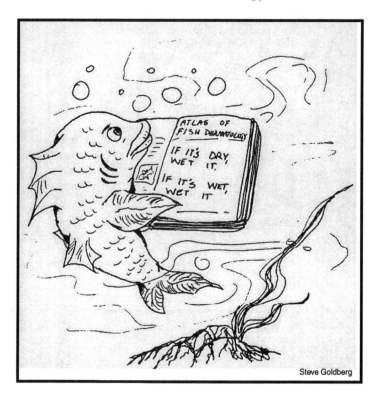

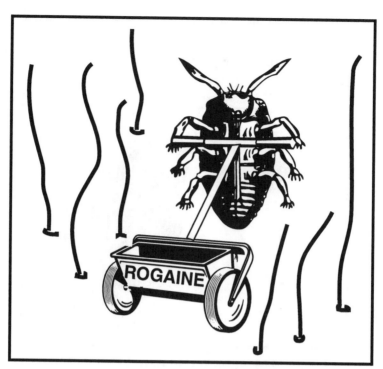

Arthur Headlouse does some home improvements.

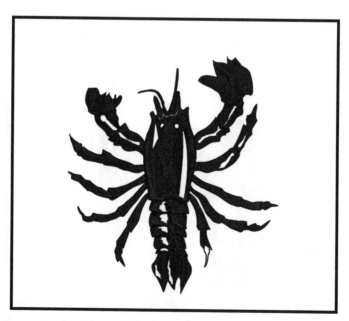

Despite all efforts, Stan's nail biting habit persisted.

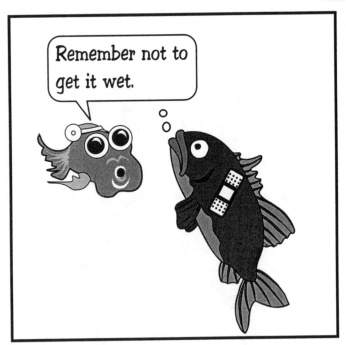

Difficult directions -- one of the major causes
of poor patient compliance.

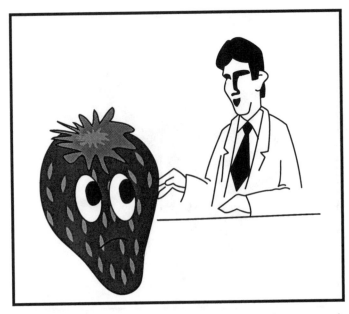

"No, its not acne, and I assure you quite normal
at your age."

DRUGS

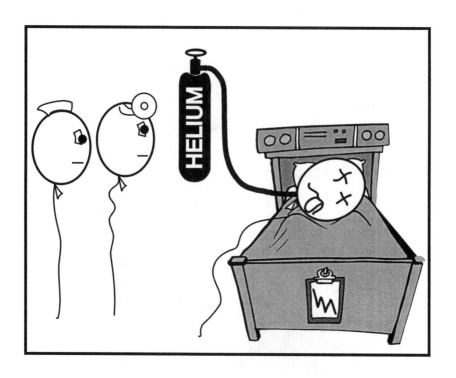

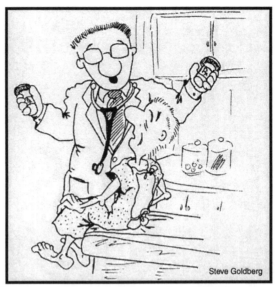

The first drug is for your high blood pressure.
The second is to counteract the first drug's
side effects, but it can increase your blood
pressure. But not to worry. If that happens,
simply take more of the first medicine.

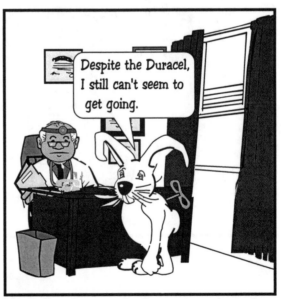

Medicine that works for one patient does
not necessarily work for another.

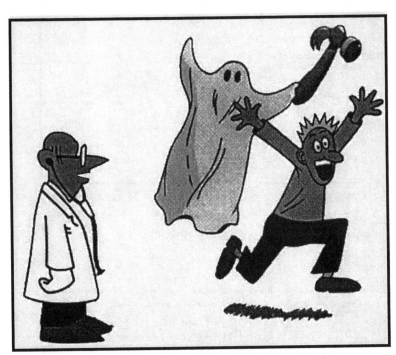

"...and if the medication causes any headaches or hallucinations, please call me."

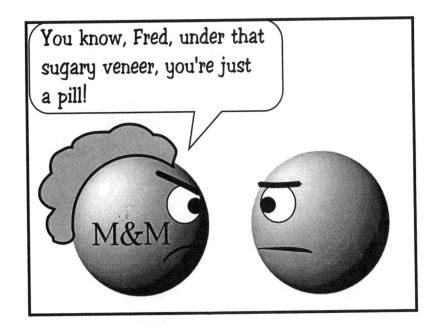

23

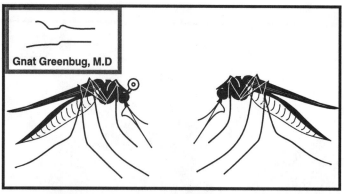

"Chemotherapy will increase your lifespan about 10 minutes, Mr. Mosley, which is not bad, given your normal life cycle of 2 days."

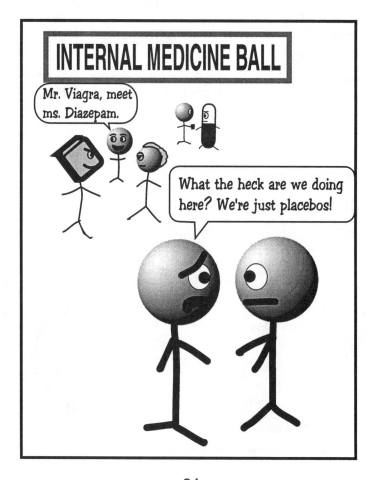

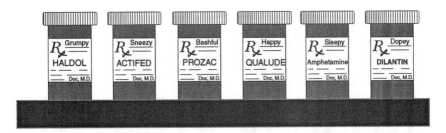

The Seven Dwarfs' medicine chest.

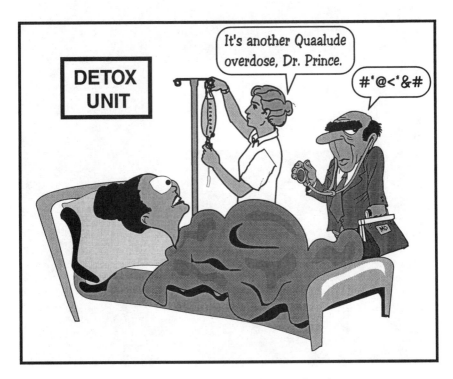

Sleeping Beauty's rude awakening

EYE, EAR, NOSE & THROAT

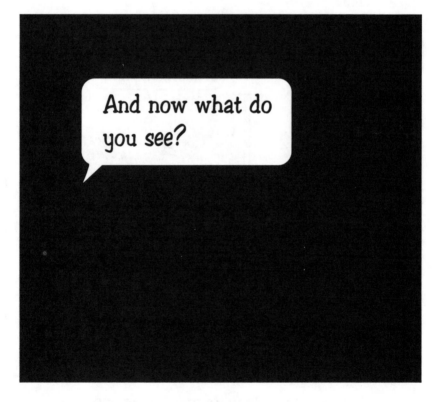

Bat visual exam

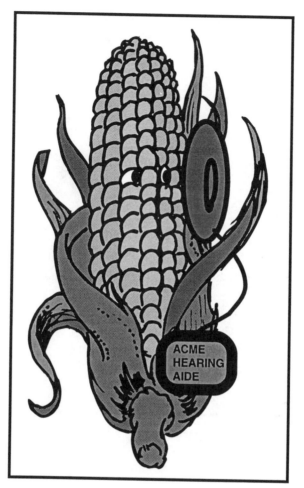

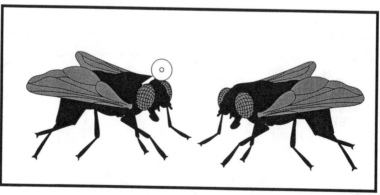

Why yes, I can operate on your cataracts. The cost will be 2 million dollars.

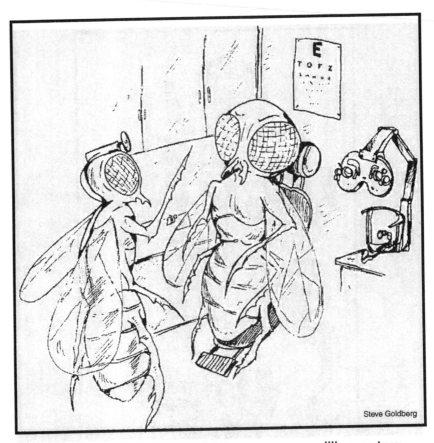

"Now how many fingers do you see, one million or two million?"

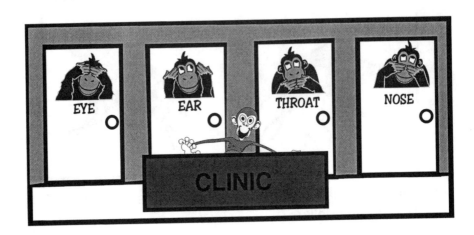

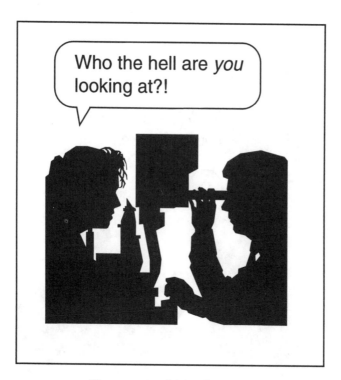

The paranoid patient.

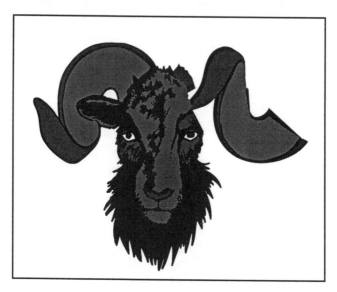

Inexpensive hearing aids.

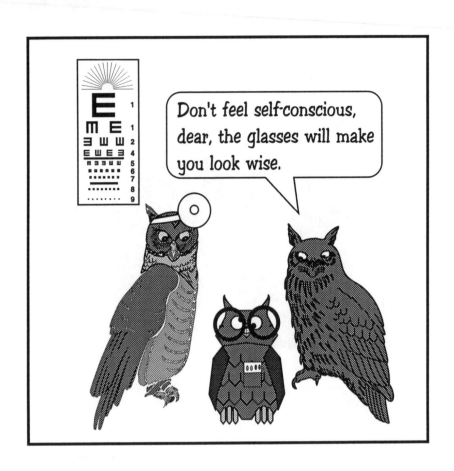

GASTROINTESTINAL

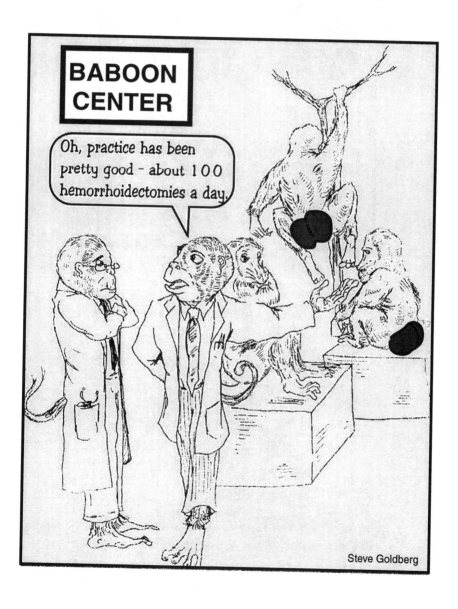

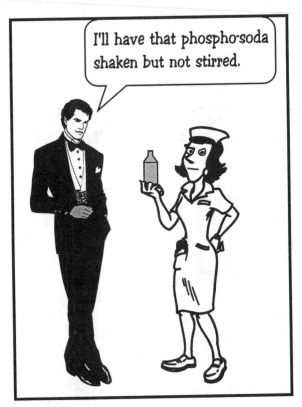

James Bond undergoes a bowel prep.

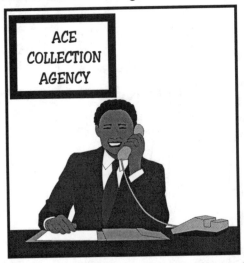

Perhaps you took me too literally, nurse Higgins. When I said we collect all kinds of crap, I was not referring to stool specimens.

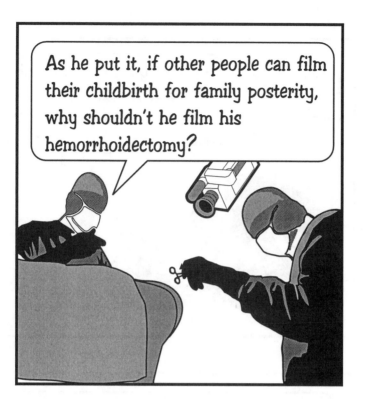

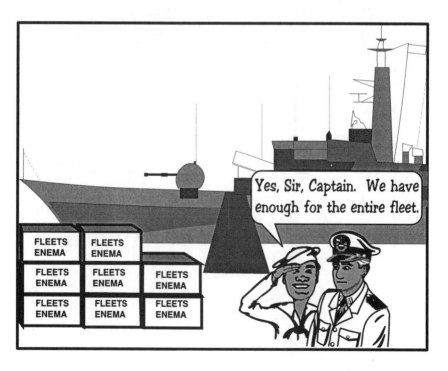

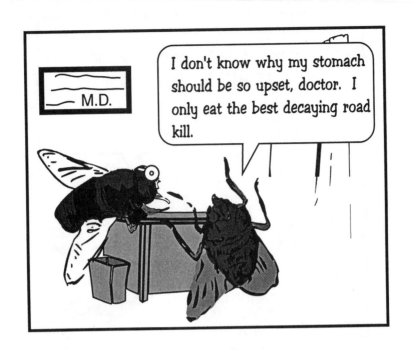

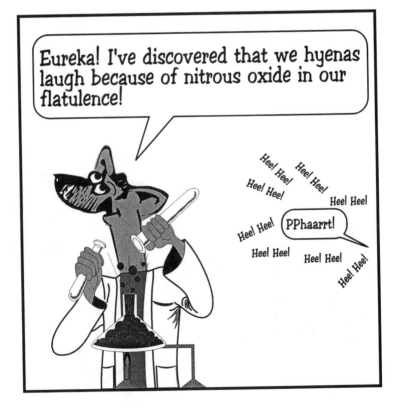

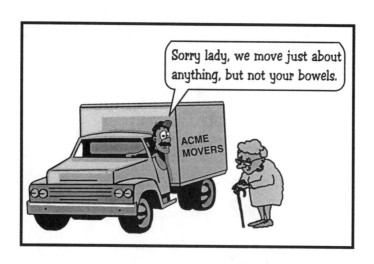

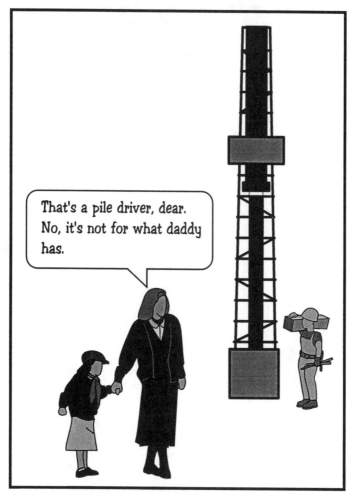

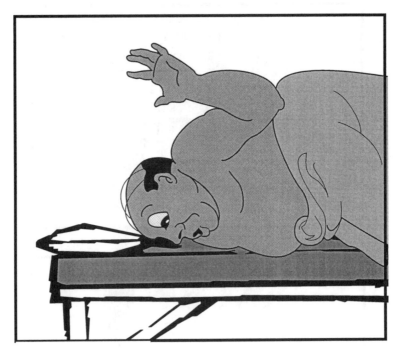

Every practitioner of Freudian psychology first has to undergo their own Sigmundoscopy.

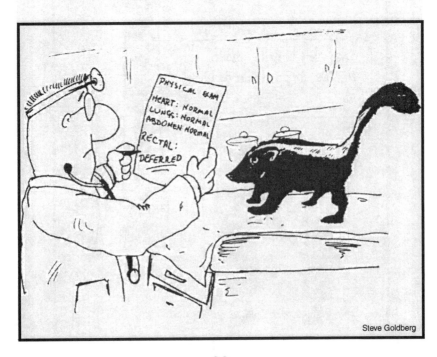

Steve Goldberg

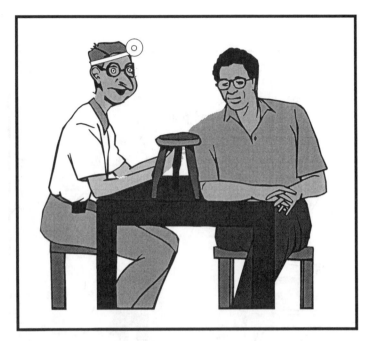

"Sorry, but that's not what I meant by a stool specimen."

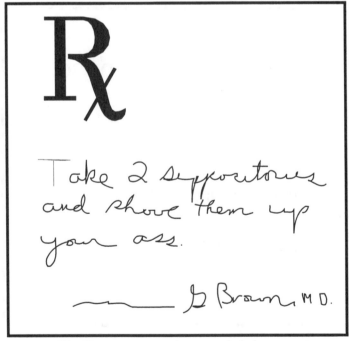

Dr. Brown experiences job burnout

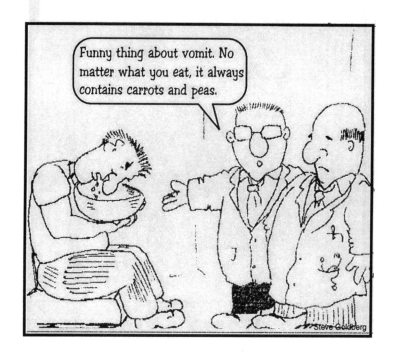

EARTHWORM SIGMOIDOSCOPY

Directions:

1. Insert in either end.

2. Look around.

INFECTIOUS
DISEASE

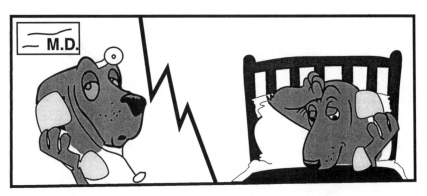

"Continue the antibiotic ...... and remember to drink lots of toilet water."

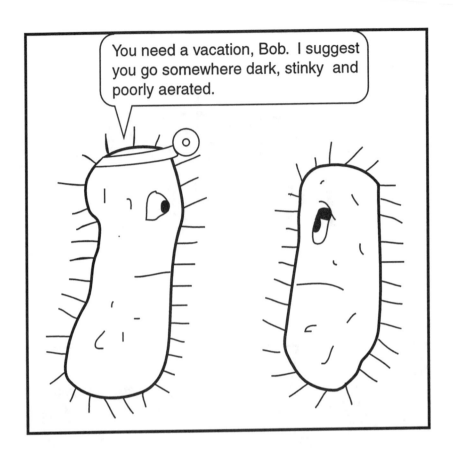

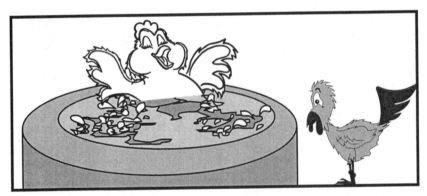

"This hot spa is great for my cold, dear . And so is the chicken soup."

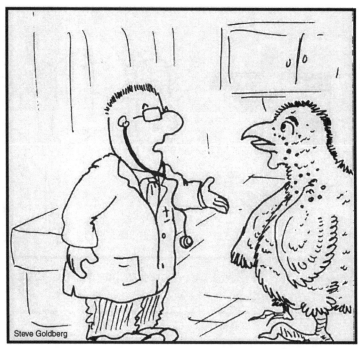

"It could be chicken pox, but then all these viruses look similar."

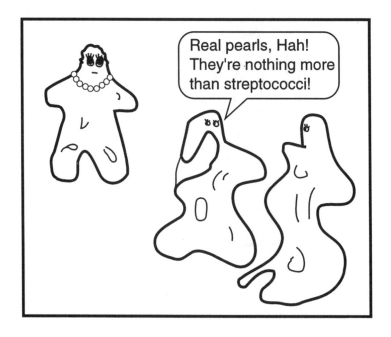

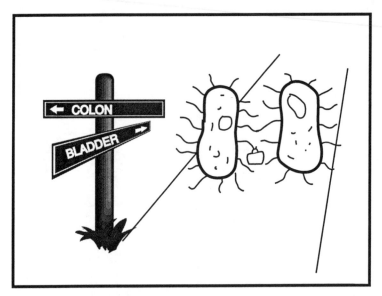

Marge and Phil leave the crowded city for the less crowded suburbs.

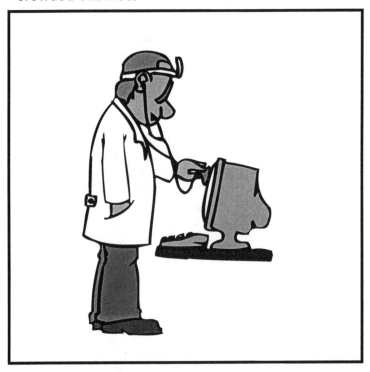

"Well, it could be a computer virus, but I think we should try an antibiotic to cover for possible bacteria."

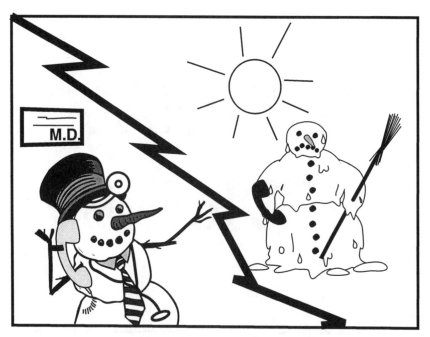

"Take two aspirin and call me in the evening."

INTERNAL

MEDICINE

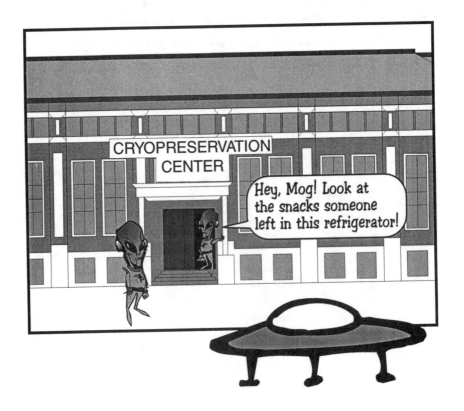

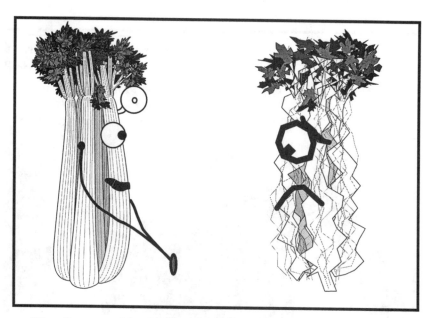

"Don't worry, Mr. Cellar, in no time I'll have you looking like a vegetable again."

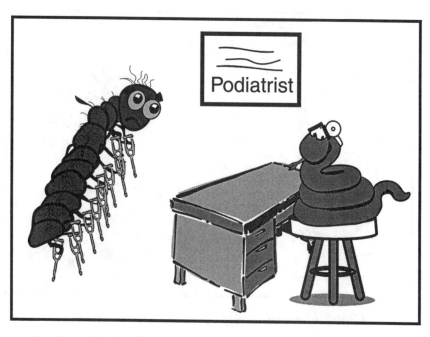

Dr. Snerkley's dismally slow practice finally takes off.

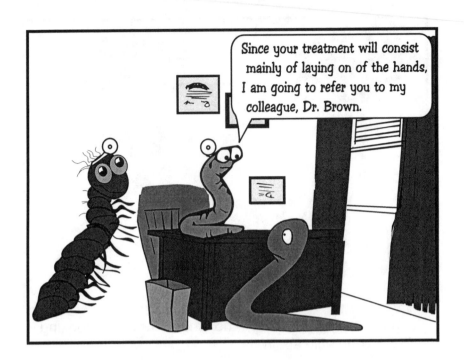

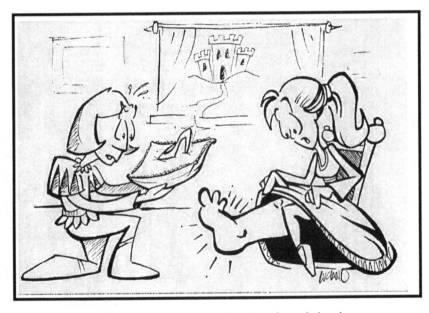

Cinderella's untimely episode of pedal edema.

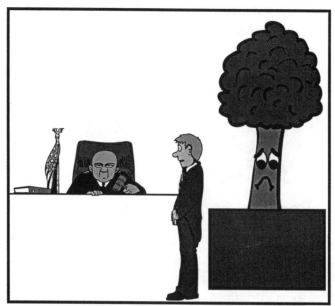

"... and so, your honor, ever since the defendant's car struck my client, she has been unable to walk."

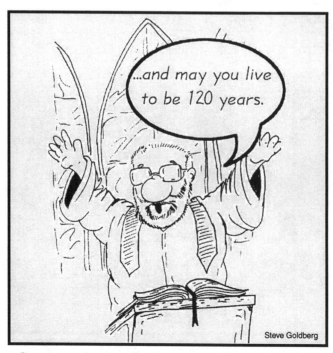

Curses - the leading cause of death in people age 120 years.

47

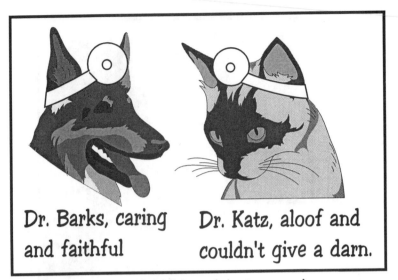

The differing personalities of doctors makes a difference in patient care.

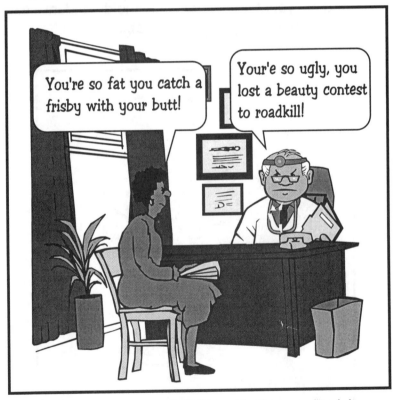

The importance of open dialogue between physician and patient.

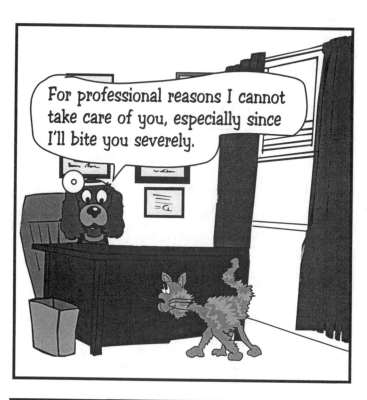

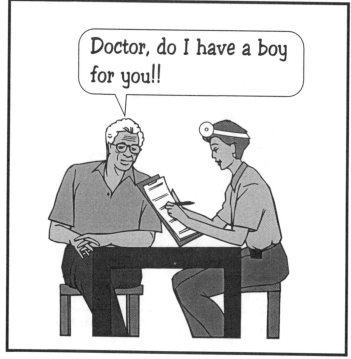

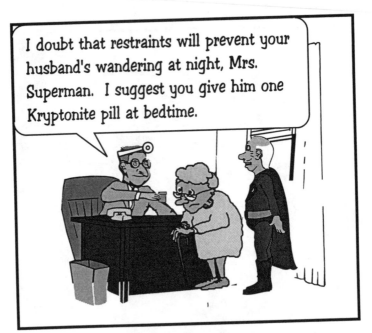

Geriatric superman

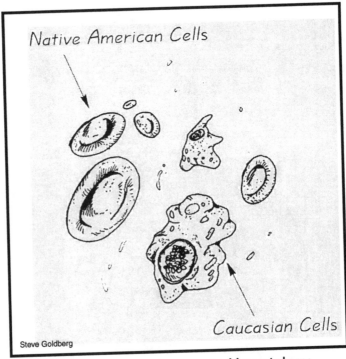

Political correctness comes to Hematology

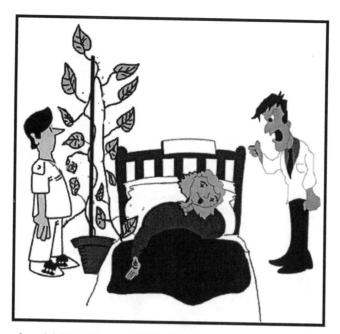

I said "Put in an IV." What could be simpler?

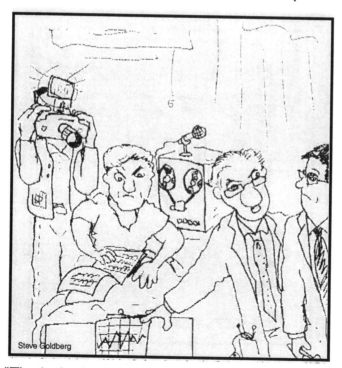

"That's the last time I treat a malpractice lawyer."

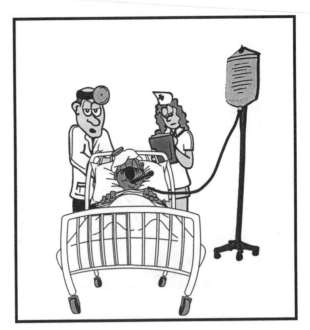

"These lucky patients, sleeping all day."

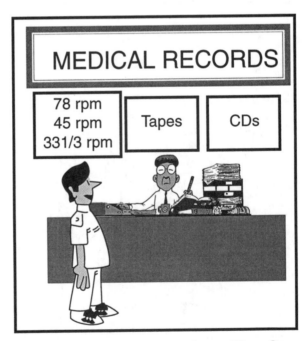

Do you have the theme music to "Ben Casey" and "E.R."?

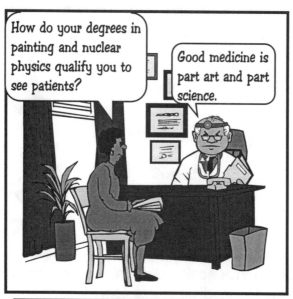

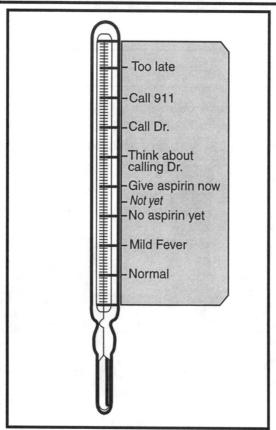

The new home thermometer.

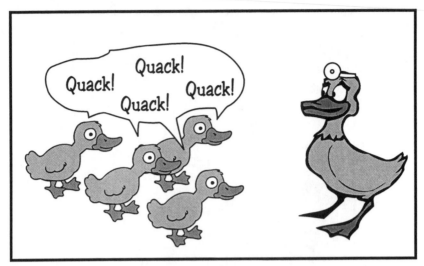

Dr Miller never achieved the respect he sought on entering the medical profession.

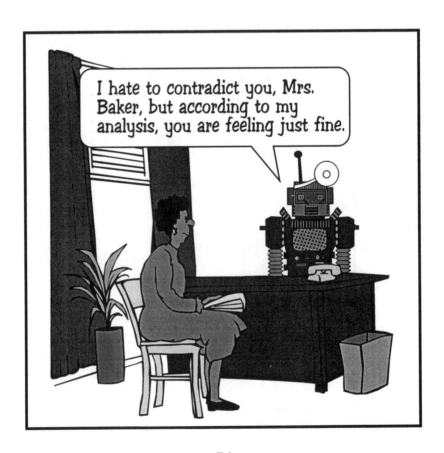

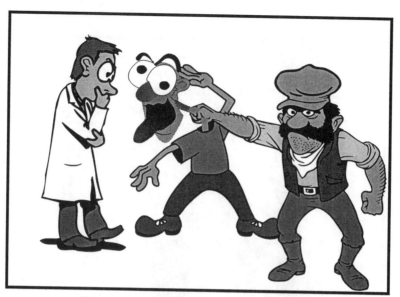

"Hmm.... could be hyperthyroidism."

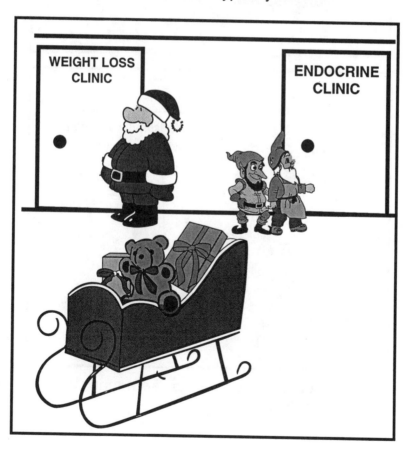

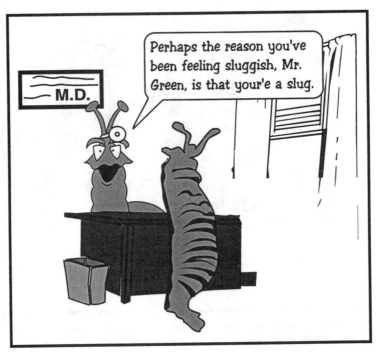

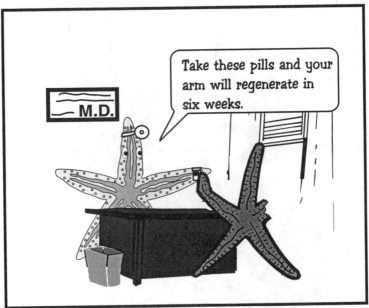

The spontaneous cure has kept many a physician in practice.

MANAGED
CARE

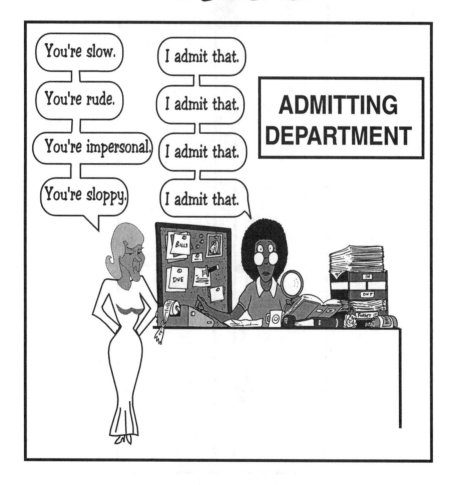

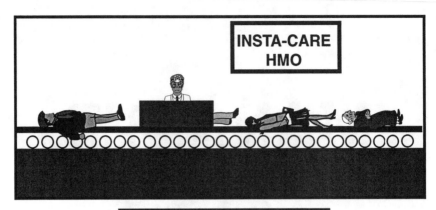

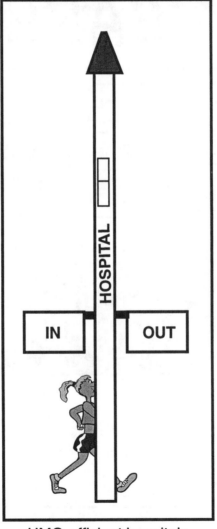

HMO-efficient hospitals

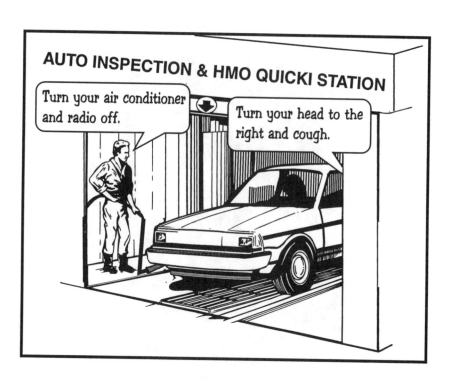

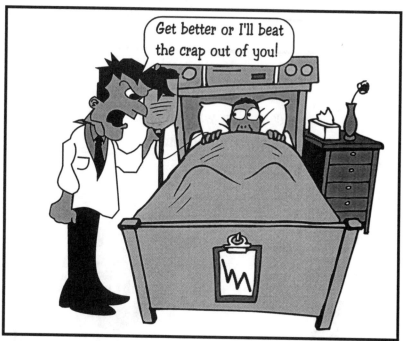

Dr. Miller tries to improve his managed care efficiency.

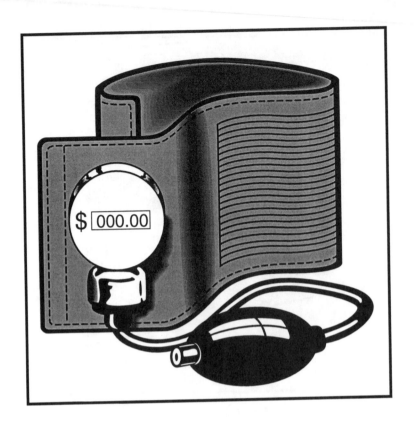

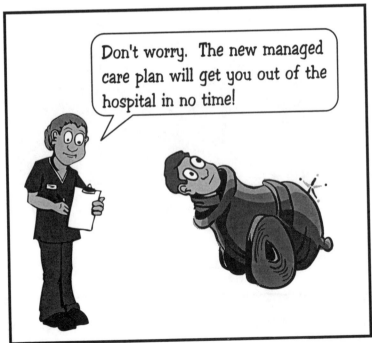

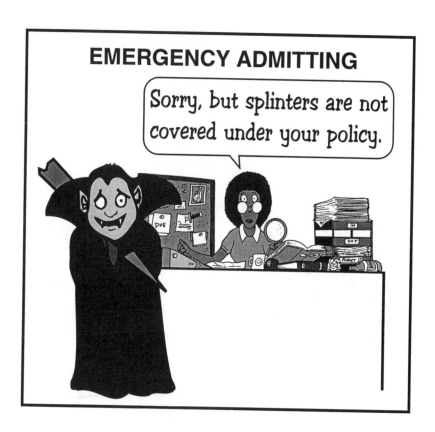

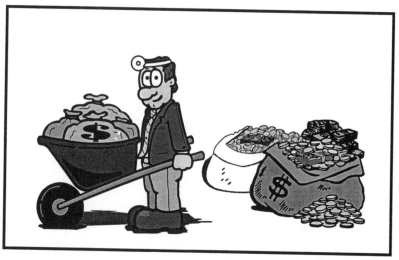

Dr. Binkley retires after performing a simple appendectomy, having "inadvertently" written the reimbursement code for an F-15 fighter.

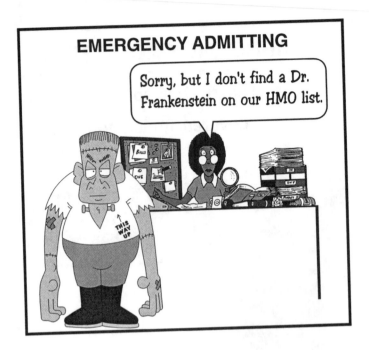

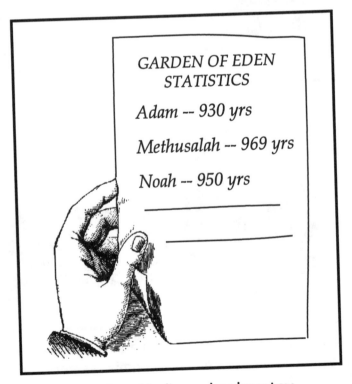

The first Medicare bankruptcy

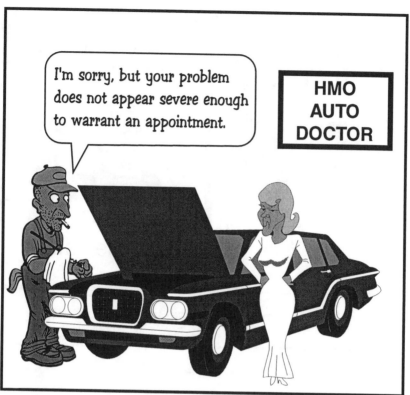

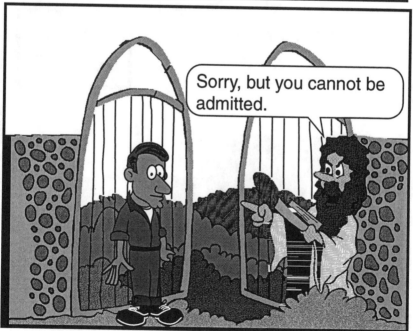

HMO Gatekeeper meets Heaven's Gatekeeper

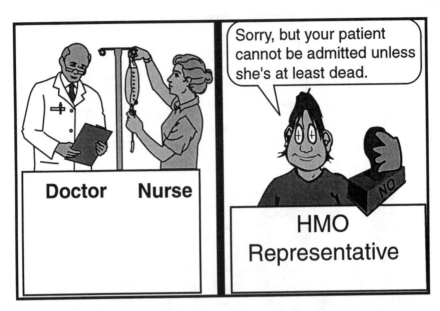

The modern medical team

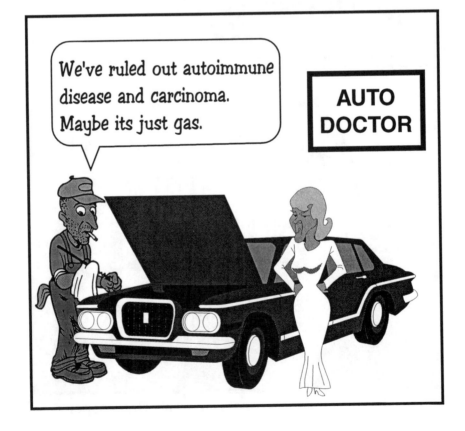

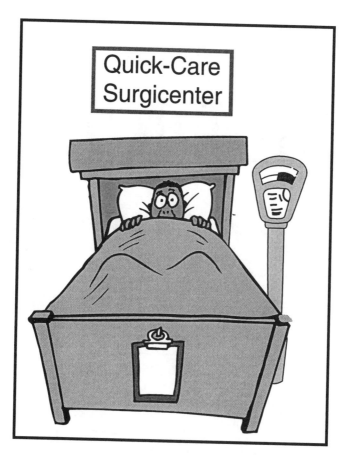

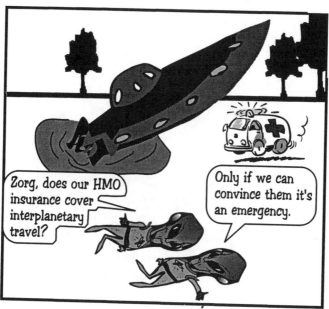

MEDICAL TRAINING

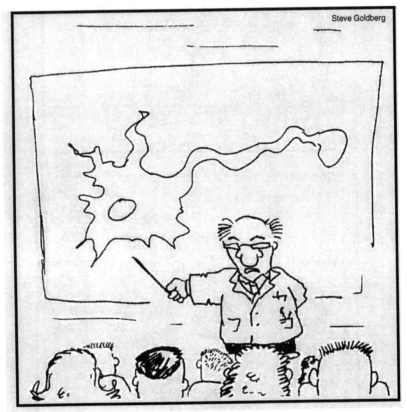

"There are 14 billion neurons in the brain and 14 billion *and one* facts to remember to pass the Boards."

ADMISSION WORKUP

Chief complaint: The patient is a 24 yo white female, about my age, who was admitted with acute onset of headache, of the sort that I have been experiencing lately.

History: The patient awoke feeling fine, much as I am feeling right now, and suddenly experienced a severe headache. Her only significant past history is that of mild hypertension, about the same level that I have been ignoring over the past few years. ...."

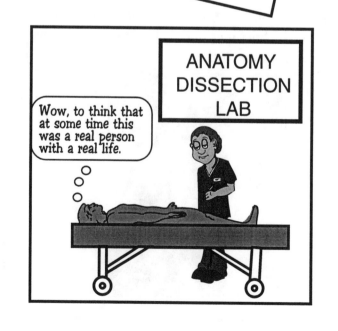

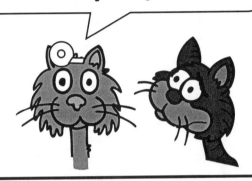

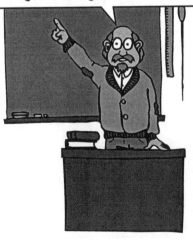

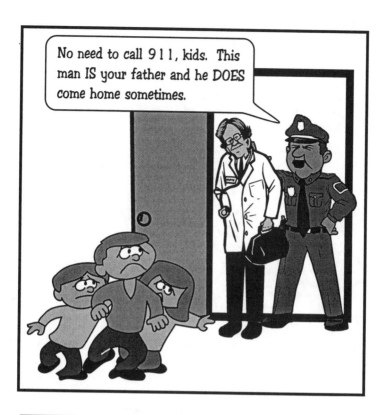

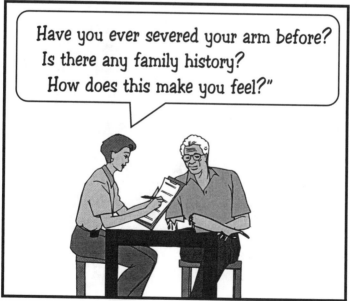

Medical student history

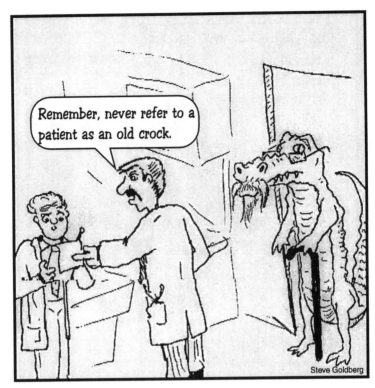

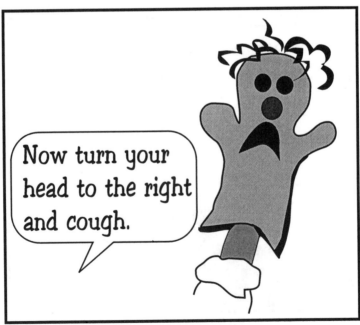

Inexpensive physical exam simulations.

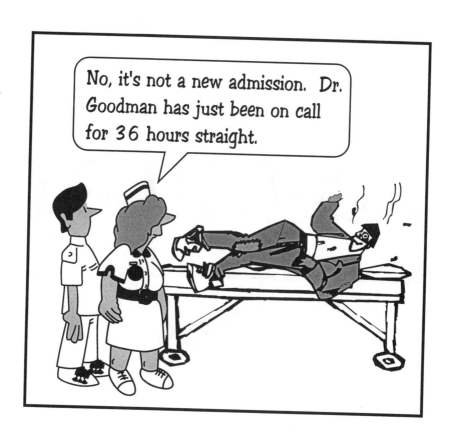

NEUROLOGY

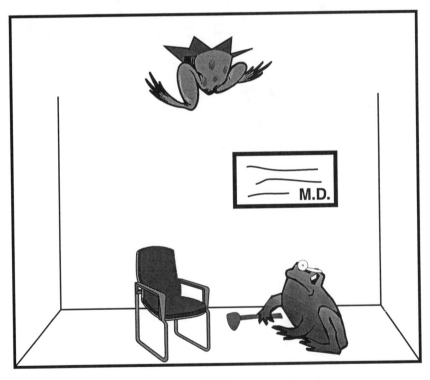

Hazards of amphibian neurology

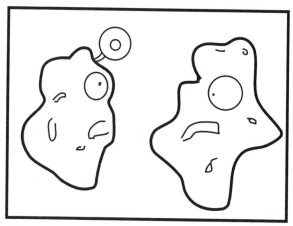

"Let me assure you Mr. Blum, you are not having a heart attack. Nor are you having pain; nor is it in you head."

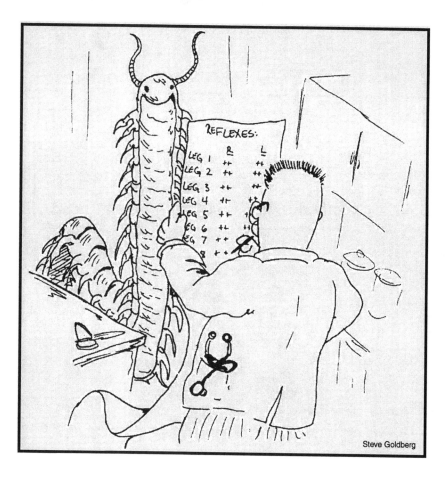

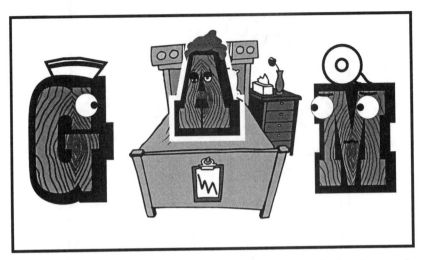

"It began with pain in her colon. Then her periods stopped, and now she's in a comma."

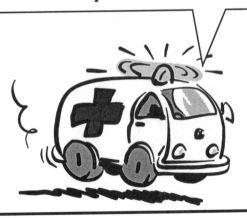

The kid Jack who fell down may have a fractured skull. The other one, Jill, says she just tumbled after. Story makes no sense. Why would one go to the TOP of a hill to fetch a pail of water?

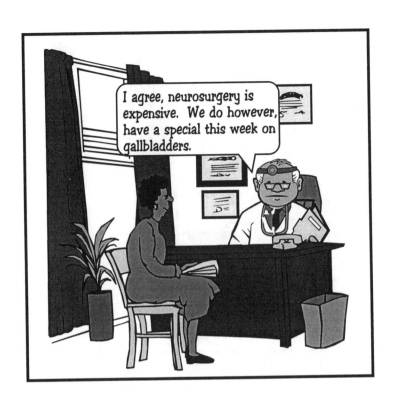

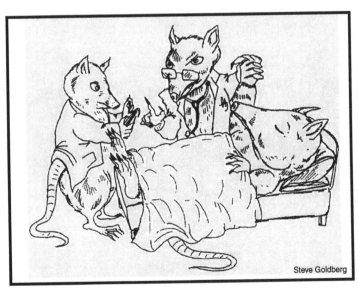

"Just drop his hand over his head. He doesn't want to hurt himself. If it hits his head, he's comatose. If it misses, he's playing possum.

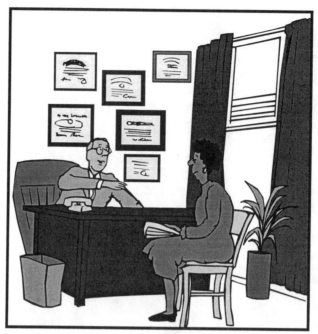

"As a professional pianist, you should know better than to play the forbidden 'spinal chord.' It sent a chill right down your spine."

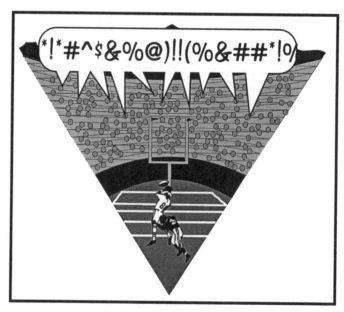

Tourette's syndrome group therapy.

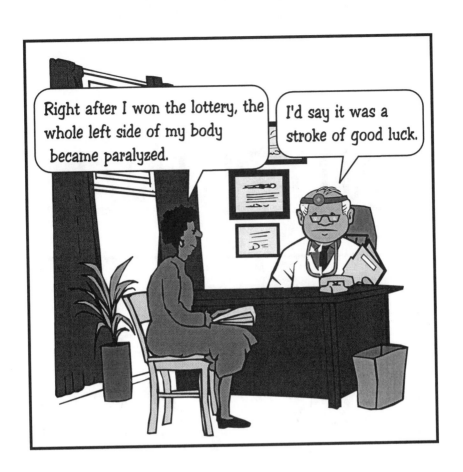

NURSING

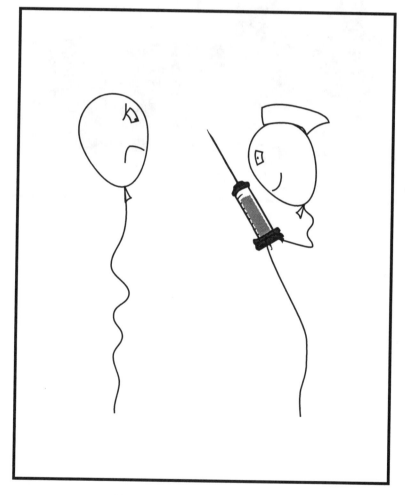

Now this won't hurt a bit

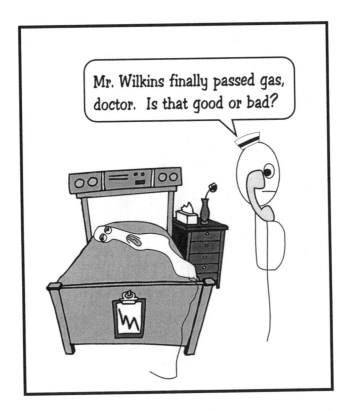

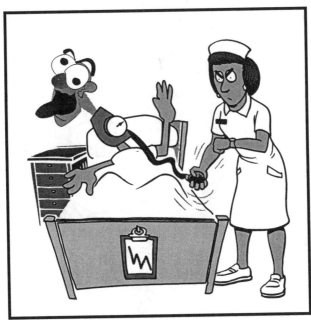

Nurse Jenkins experiences job burnout.

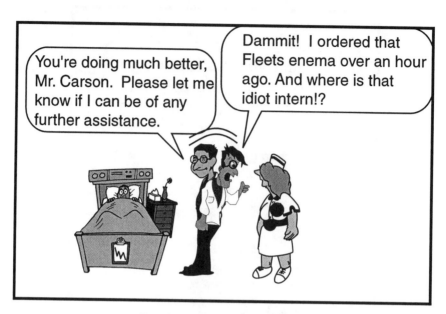

Dr. Jeckyl and Dr. Hyde

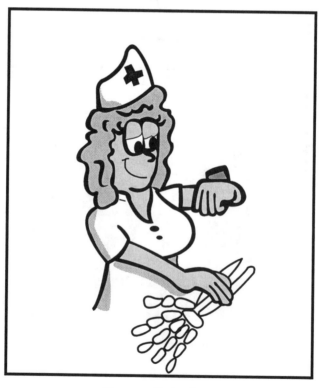

Easy admission

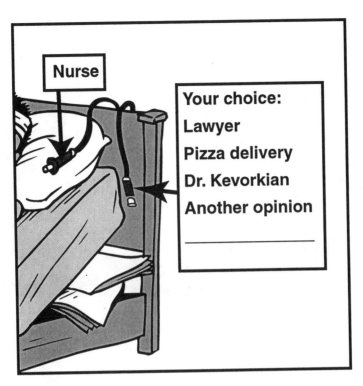

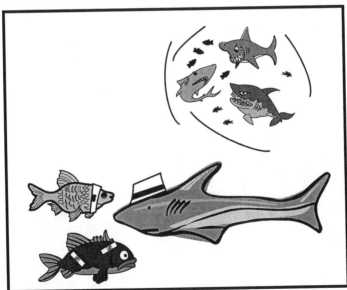

The nurse shark, heroine of the feeding frenzy battlefield.

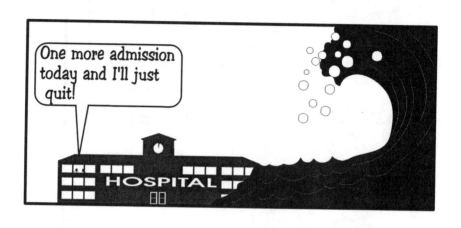

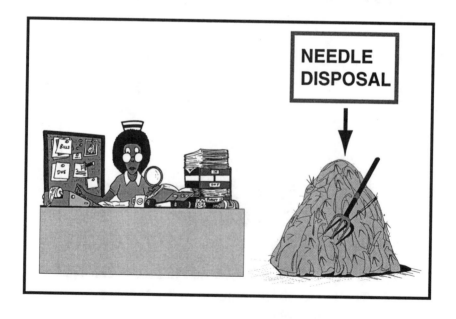

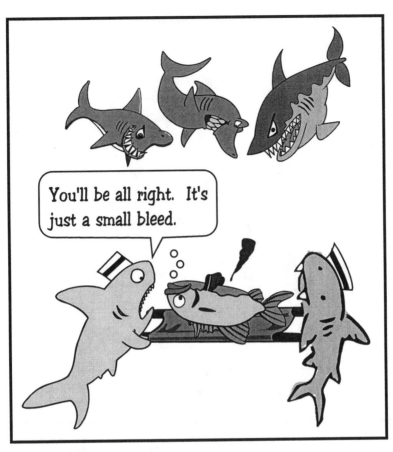

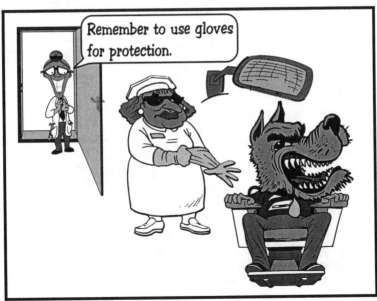

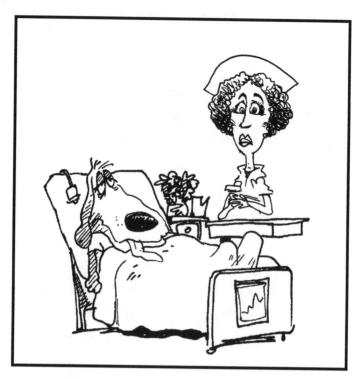

"Nurse, may I have the tree please."

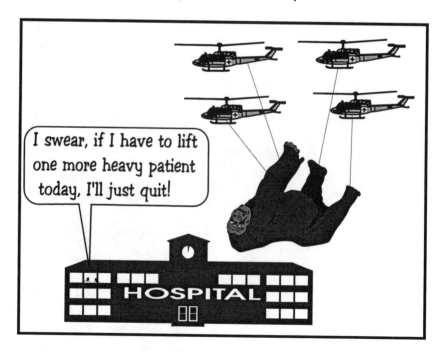

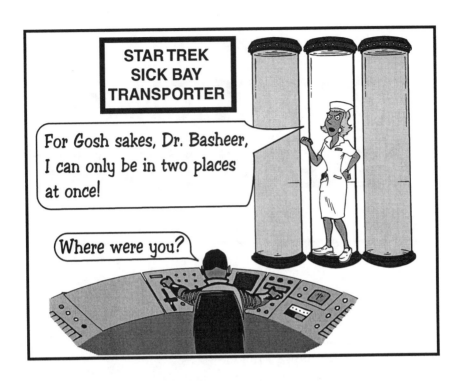

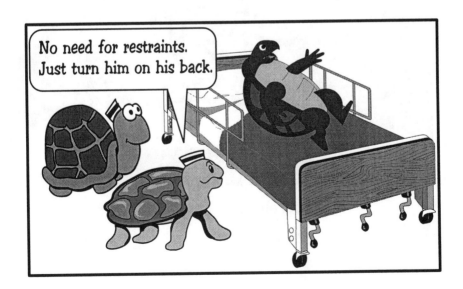

NUTRITION & GENERAL HEALTH

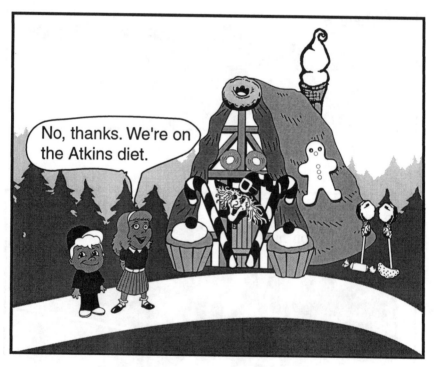

Hansel and Gretel luck out.

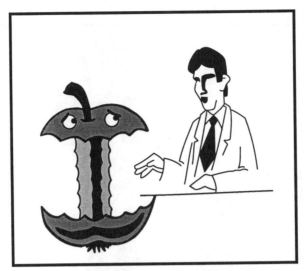

"Well, I'm not totally sure, but you either have anorexia or bulemia."

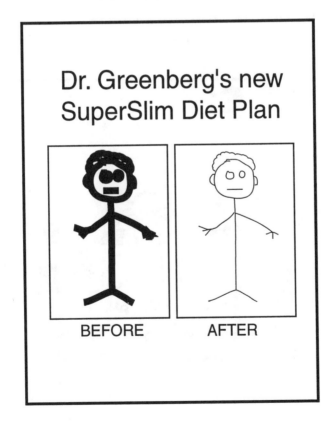

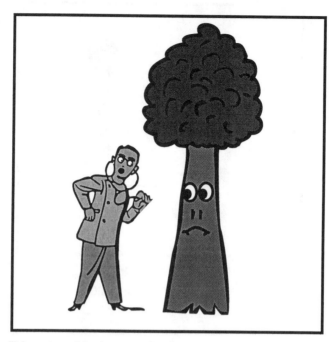

"Your trouble is you don't get enough exercise"

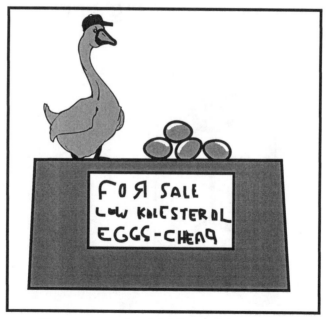

FOR SALE
LOW KOLESTEROL
EGGS-CHEAP

The goose who laid the golden eggs --
talented, but not business savvy.

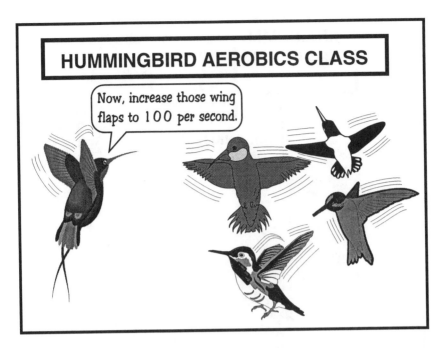

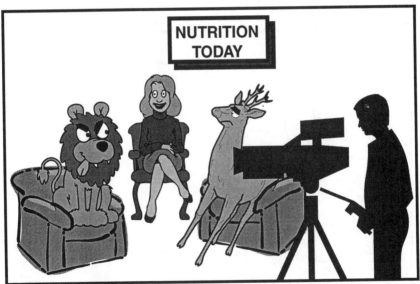

"--and today's panelists are Dr. Hugh Lions and Dr. Dawn Deerfield, who will debate the pros and cons of a meat versus vegetarian diet."

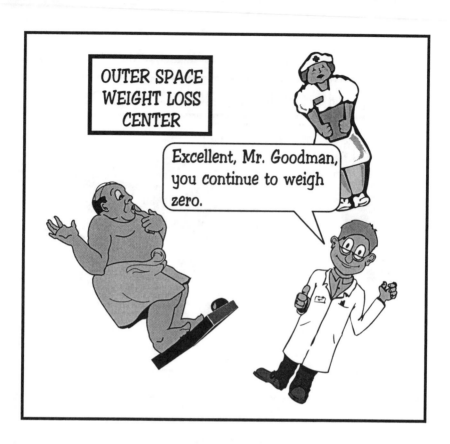

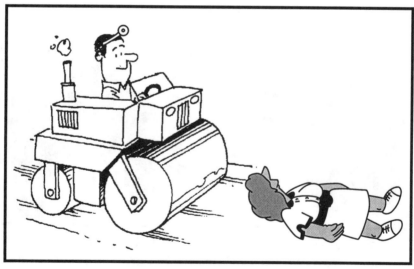

Dr. Gilbert's Five-Second Weight Loss Plan

OB/GYN

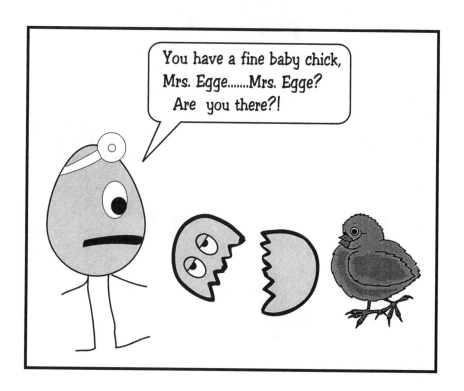

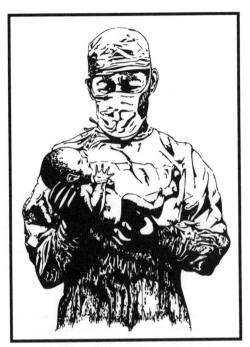

AT & T's new cordless delivery.

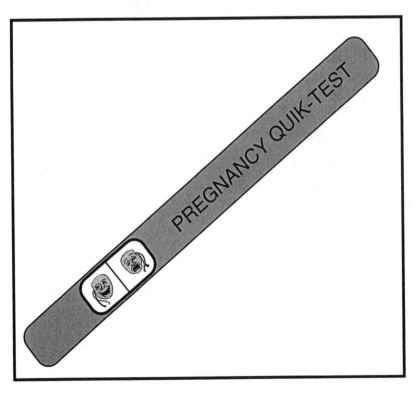

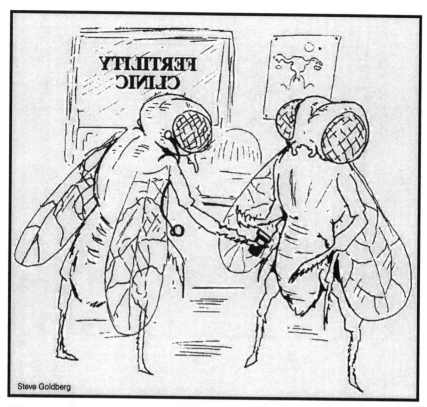

These pills should help, Mrs. Gordon, but you might lay up to 20,000 eggs.

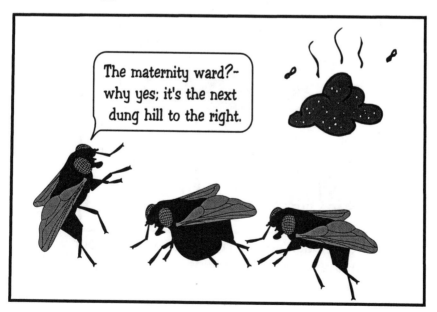

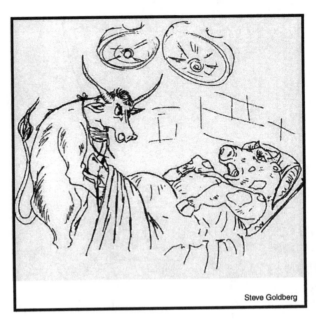

"Relax, Mrs. Benson, don't have a cow."

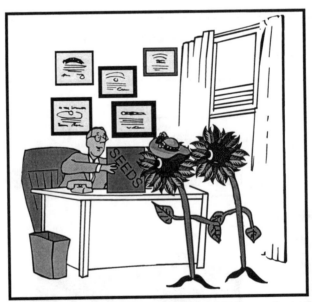

"Even though you can't have children of your own, there are other options. Try planting some of these."

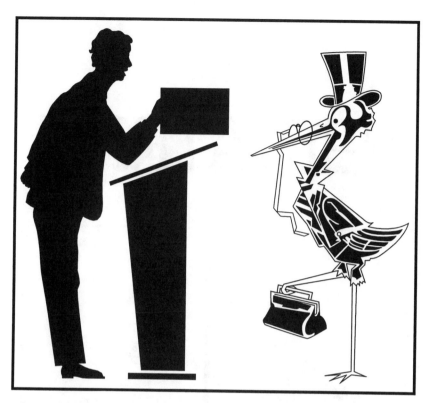

Once, again, Dr. Cramer receives the "Low-Caesarean Rate of the Year" award.

PEDIATRICS

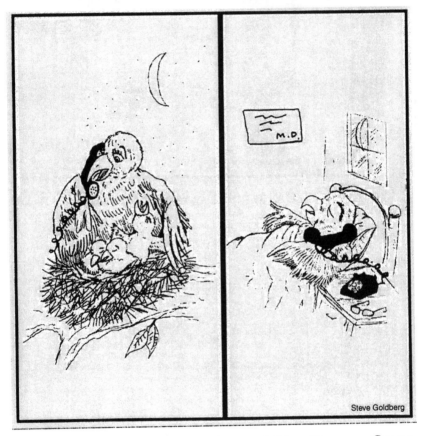

Steve Goldberg

"Just keep feeding them on demand, Mrs. Rogers. Some children need more than others.

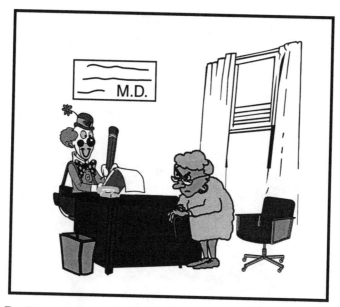

Dr. Hammerman discovers that the change from pediatric to geriatric practice is not that simple.

PEDIATRIC LAB REPORT

PATIENT: Allison Brown   AGE: 9

SUGAR: 107

SPICE: 7.9

EVERYTHING NICE: 139

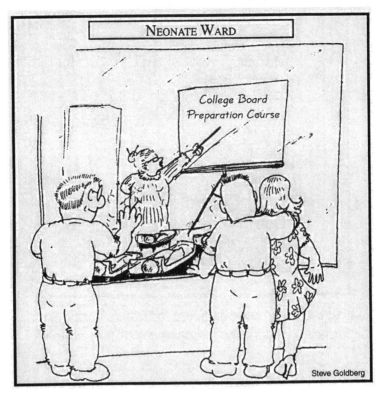

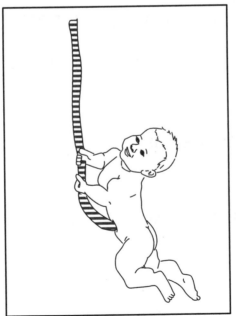

Neonatal Arnold Schwartzenegger
starts his workout training early.

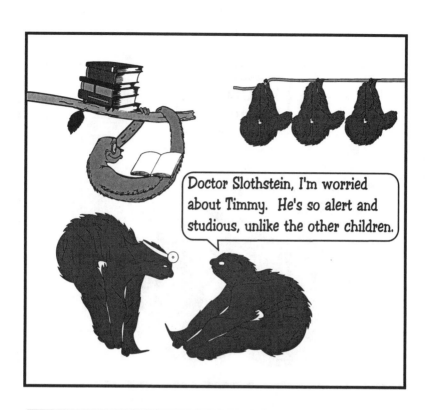

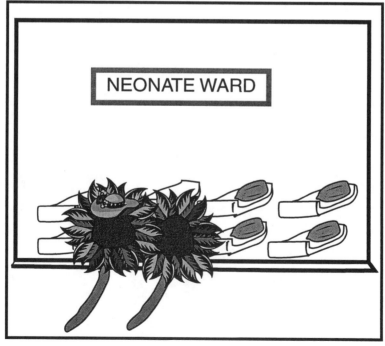

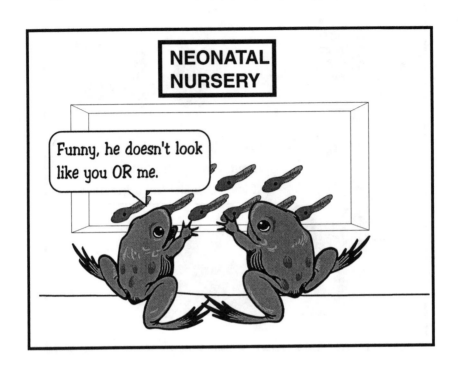

PSYCHIATRY

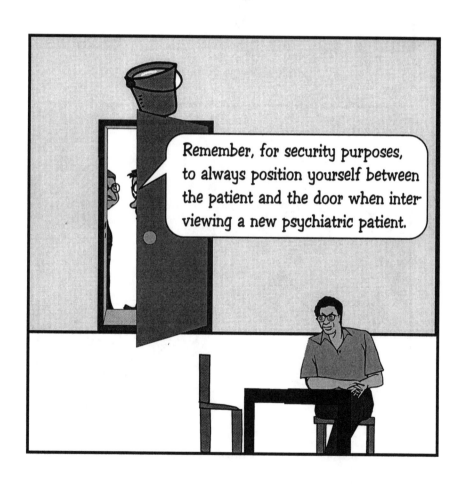

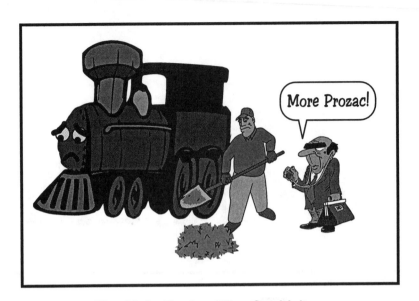

The Little Engine Who Couldn't

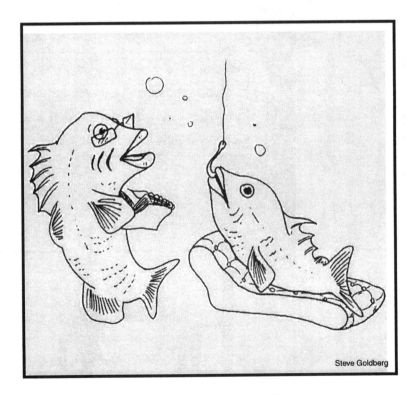

"And how long have you been feeling that people are after you?"

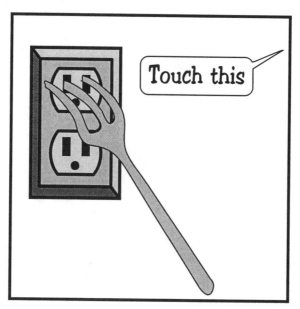

Low cost electroconvulsive therapy

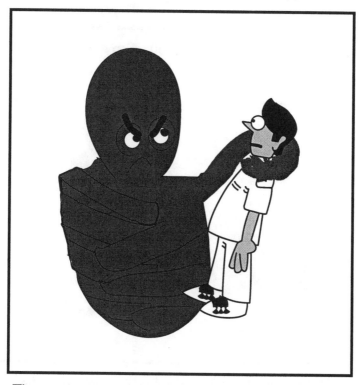

The octopus straight jacket -- not yet perfected.

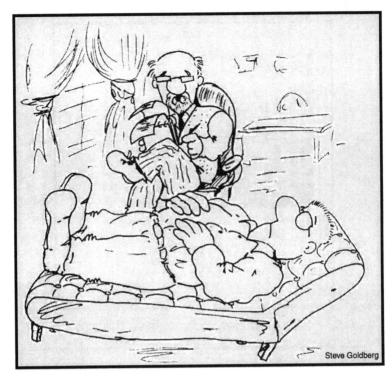

"And how long have you been, in my opinion, evil?"

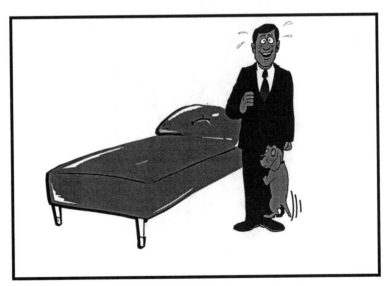

Dr. Ginsberg, animal psychiatrist, experiences doctor-patient transference.

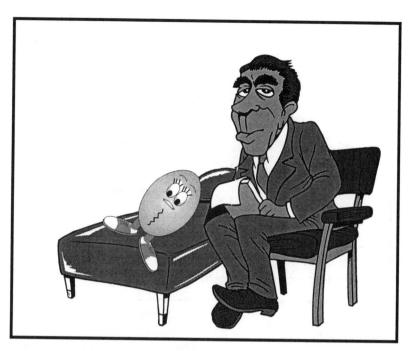

"...and every since my pregnancy, I've felt like an empty shell."

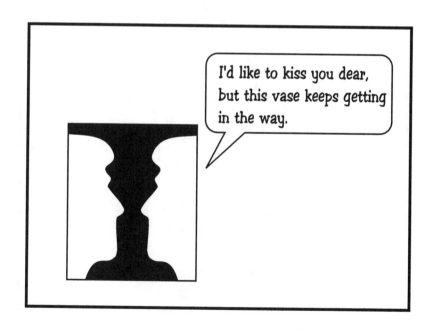

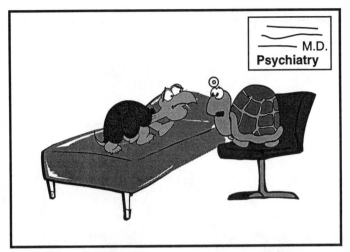

"Anytime a difficult situation arises, I suggest you simply withdraw into your shell, rather than facing it."

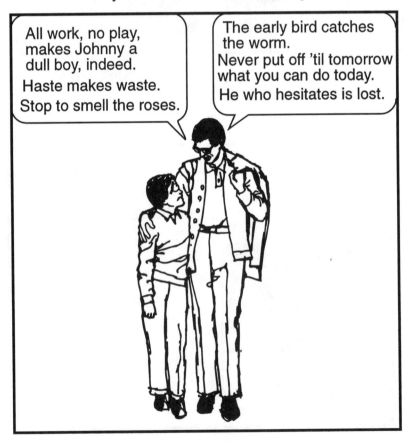

The tragedy of parental inconsistency.

RADIOLOGY

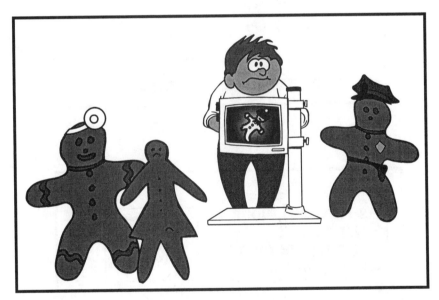

Don't worry, Mrs. Gingerbread. We'll find a way to get your son out somehow.

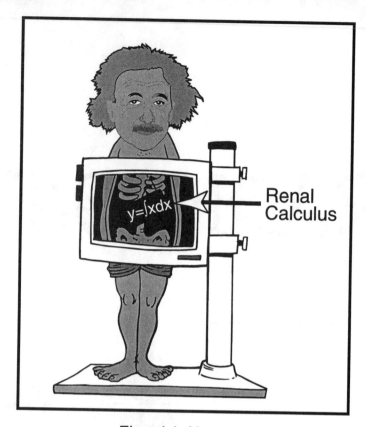

Einstein's X-ray

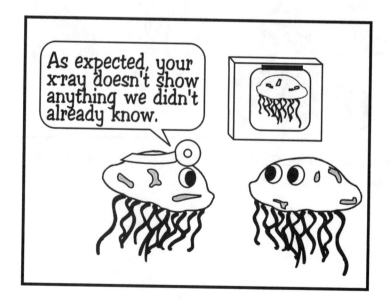

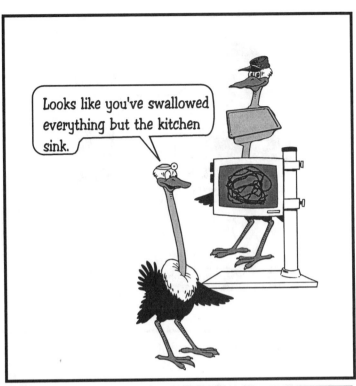

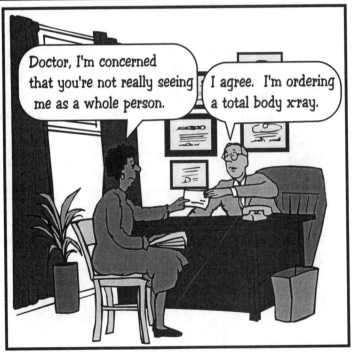

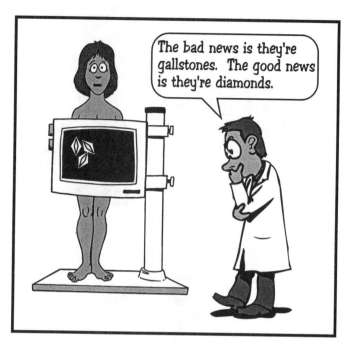

Diseases of the rich.

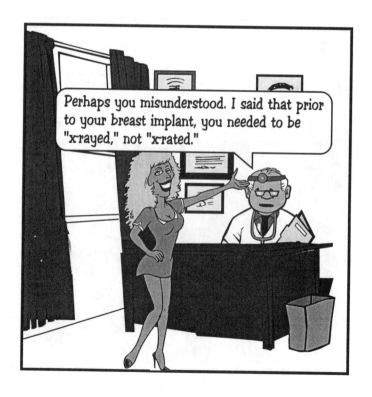

SEX &
MARRIAGE
CONSELING

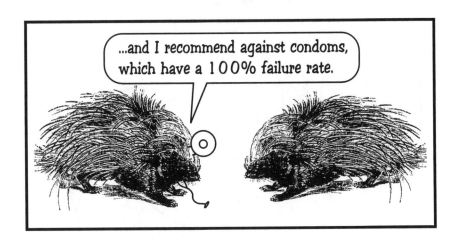

...and I recommend against condoms, which have a 100% failure rate.

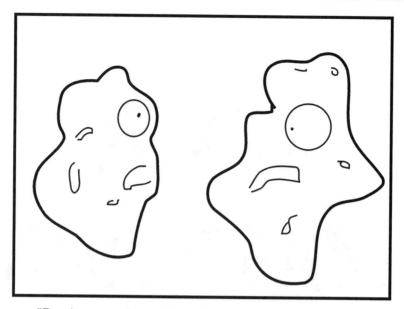

"Don't worry Dear, Erectile dysfunction isn't the end of the world, especially if you're an ameba."

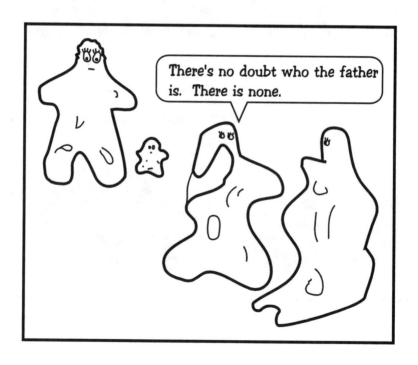

There's no doubt who the father is. There is none.

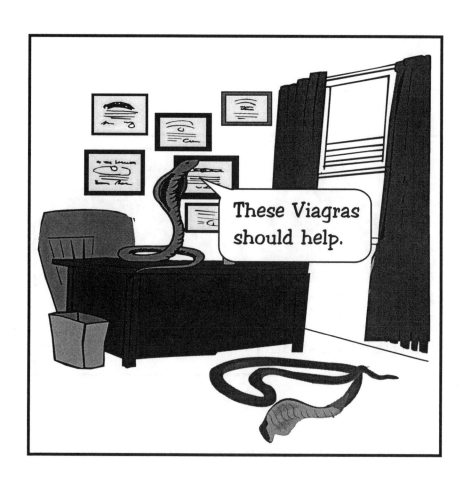

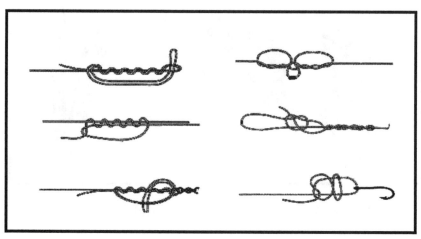

Earthworm Kama Sutra

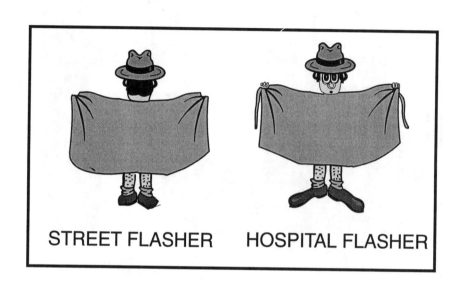

STREET FLASHER   HOSPITAL FLASHER

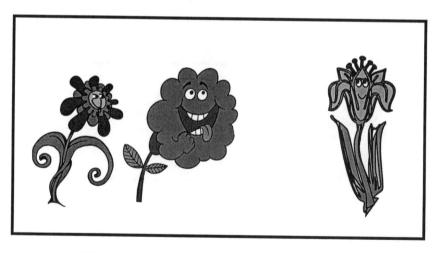

"Wow! Look at the pistils on that Babe!"

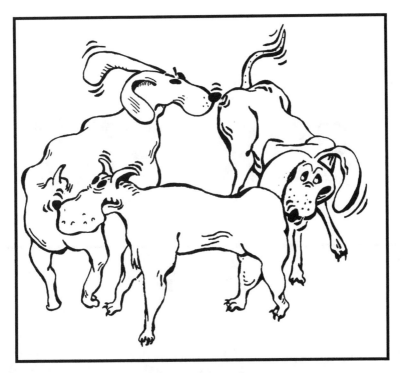

Menage a trois

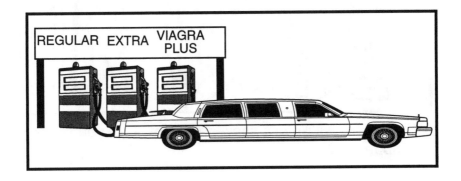

SURGERY

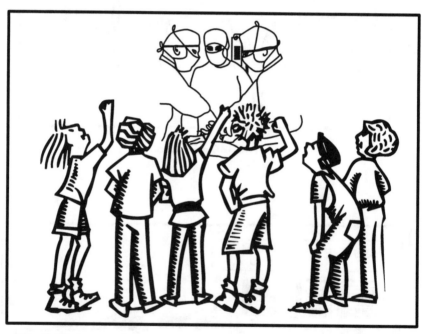

"Excuse us, we're on a scavenger hunt. Can you spare an appendix?"

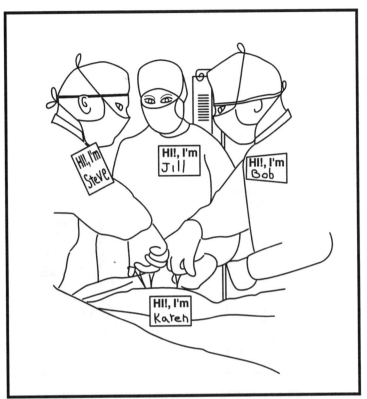

Adding the human touch to the operating room.

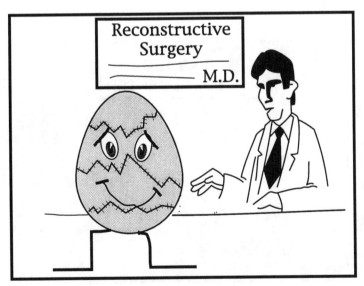

"I'm glad you didn't just rely on horses and King's men, Mr. Dumpty."

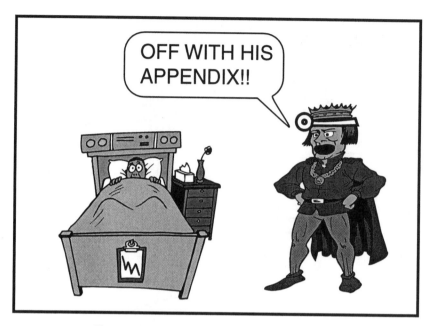

Ego problems on the surgical service

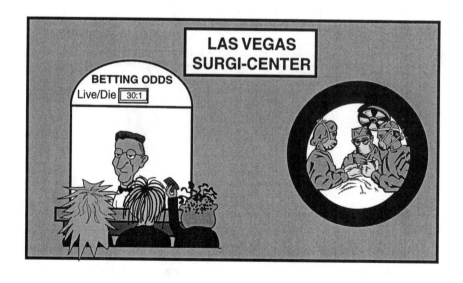

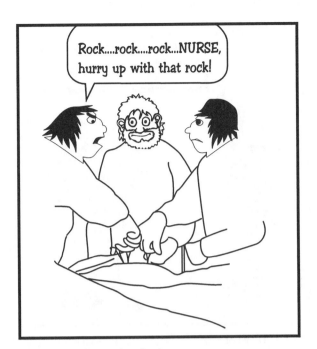

Neanderthal surgery

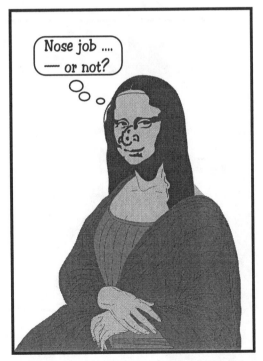

Mona Lisa's fateful career decision.

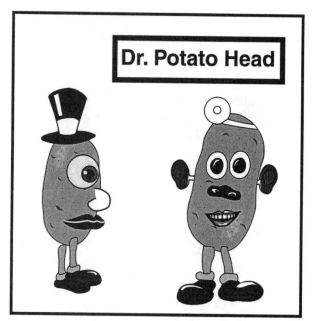

I'm running a special on facial reconstructive surgery today. Only 25 cents.

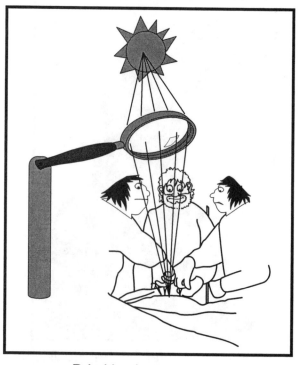

Primitive laser surgery

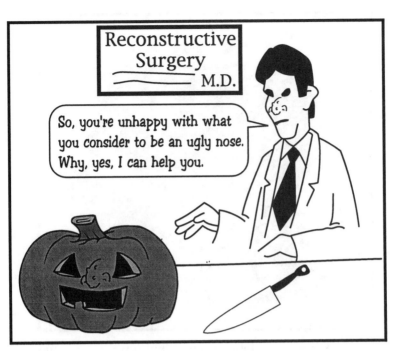

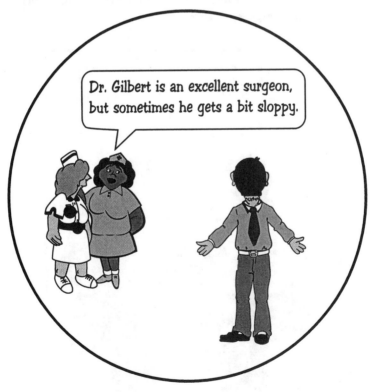

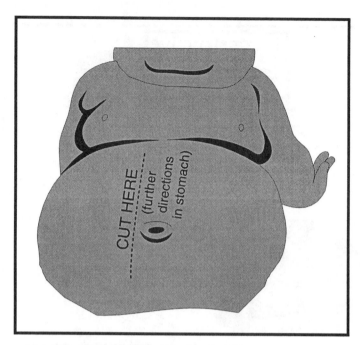

Mrs. Higgins insisted on participating in her own medical decision-making.

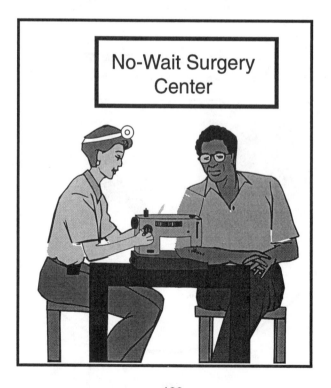

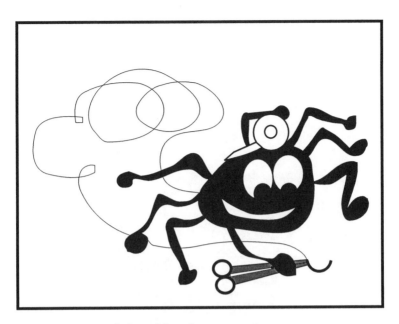

8-0 spiderchrome sutures

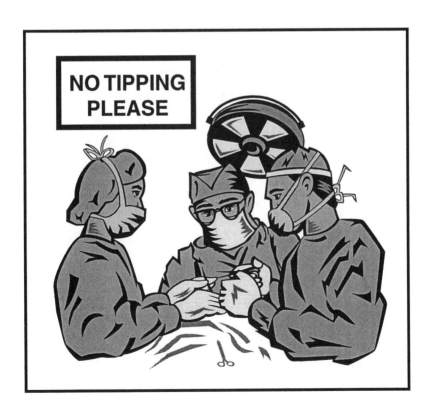

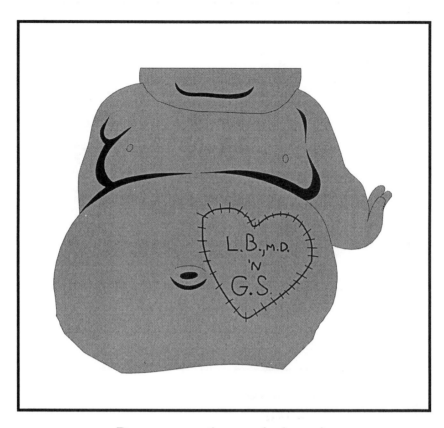

Romance on the surgical service

TRAUMA

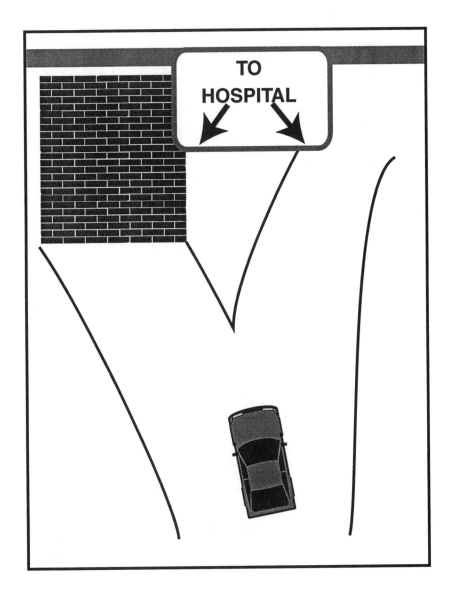

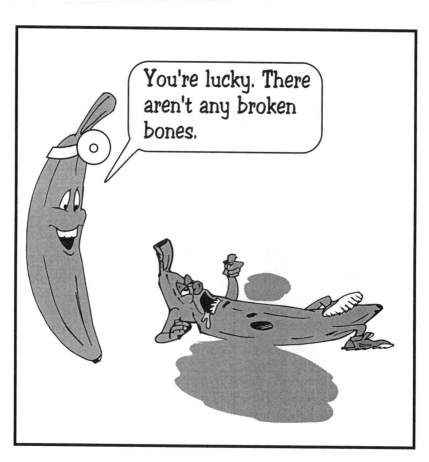

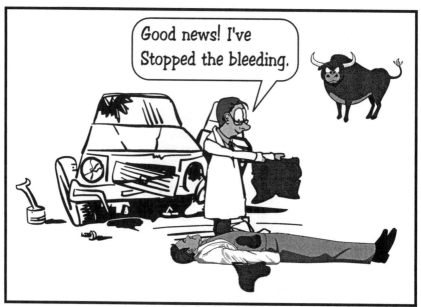

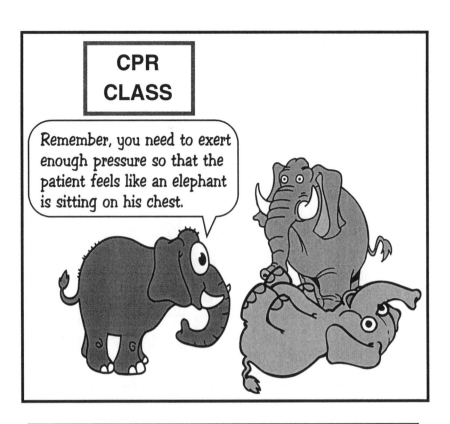

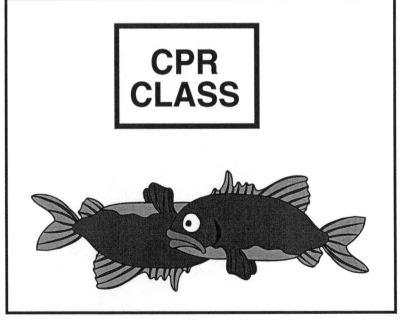

Gill-to-gill resuscitation

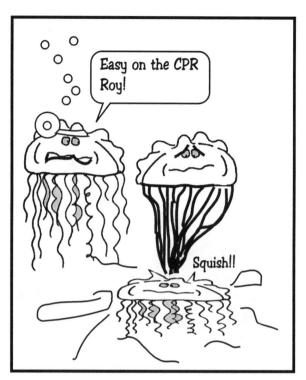

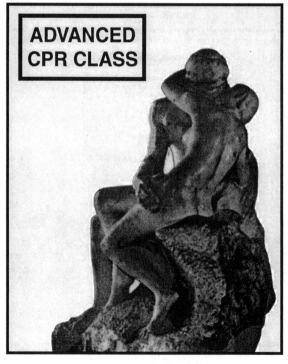

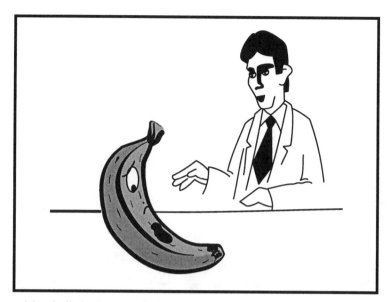

It's definitely a soft tissue injury. Have you, by any chance been living in the refrigerator?"

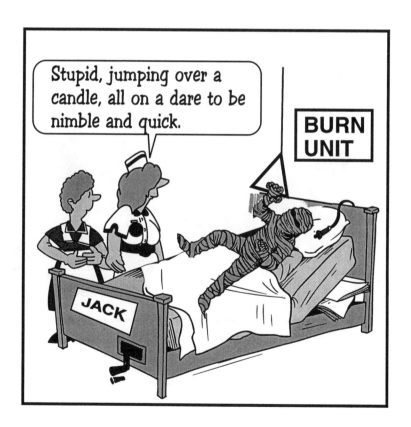

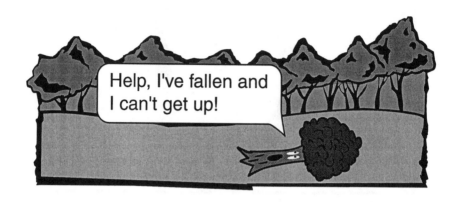

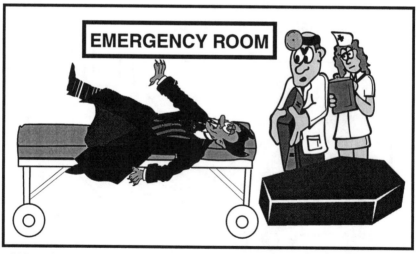

"Now how could he have type A, B, AB, O, Rh- *AND* Rh+ on the type and cross match?"

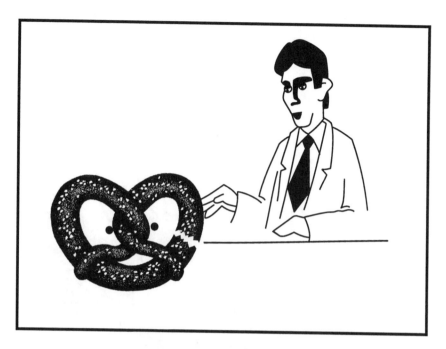

"Well, I think splinting will help, but frankly I don't think it will ever heal completely."

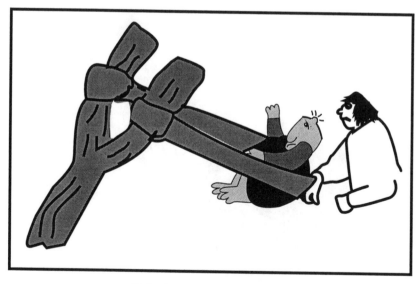

Primitive ambulances.

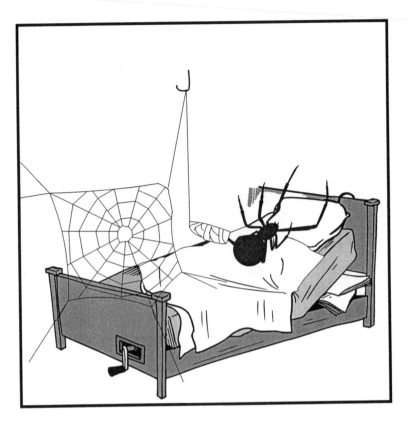

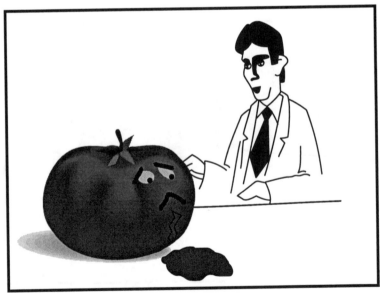

"Relax. It's not blood. It's just ketchup."

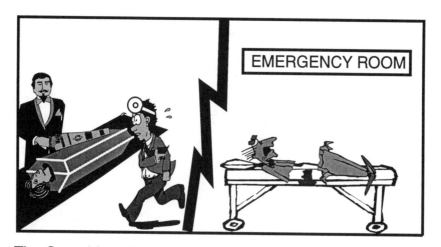

The Great Magnifico is called for an emergency consultation.

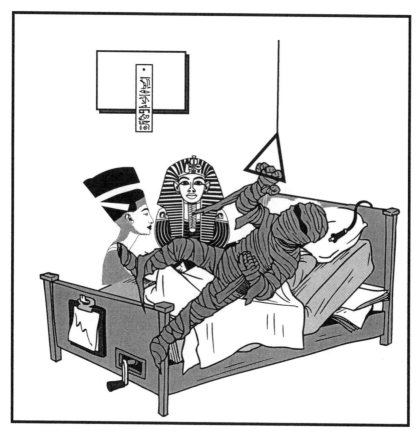

"I'm not Akhanatan, I'm Jerry Smith, and where are my skis?"

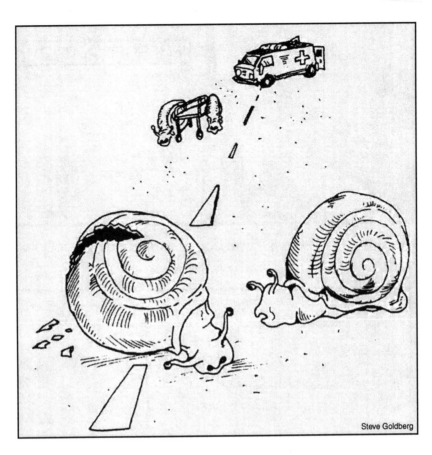

Easy, John, help will be here any day now.

UROLOGY

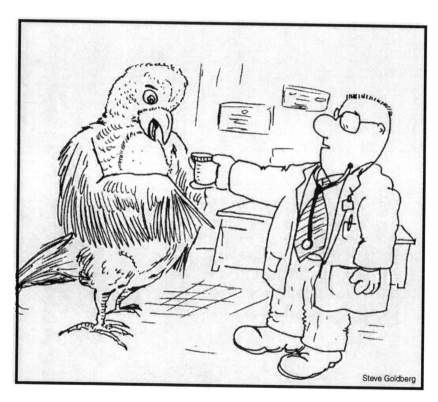

"What's a urine specimen?"

Steve Goldberg

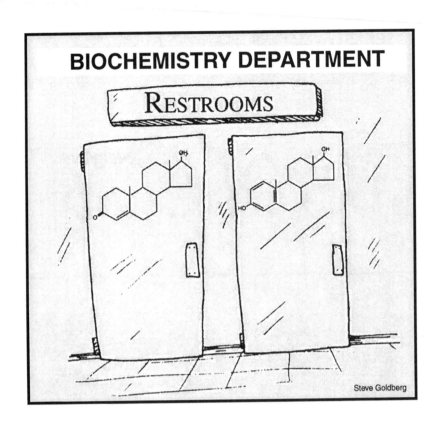

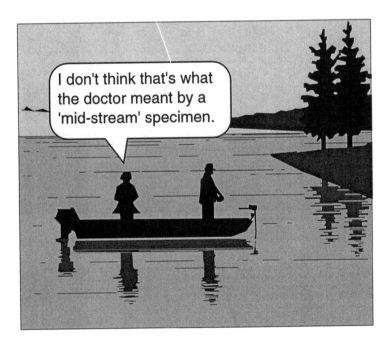

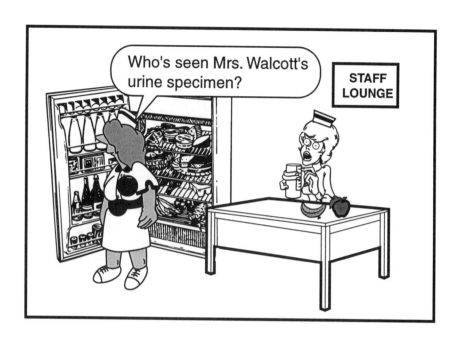

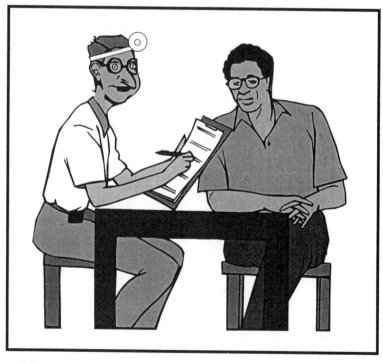

"Your failure to experience pain in the genital region is the well-known condition 'penopainopenia'."

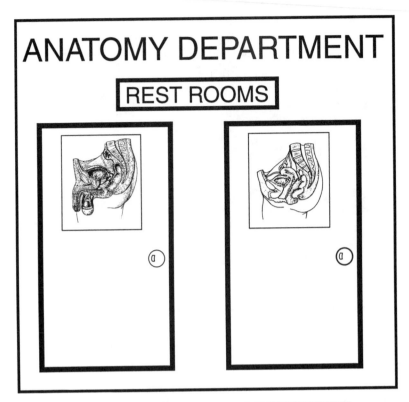

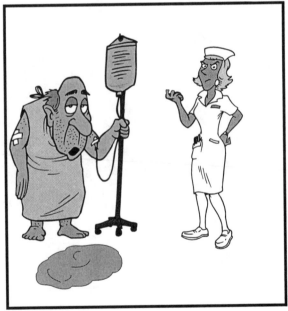

"What's wrong with peeing on the floor. I got this
contest coupon that says '*Void Where Prohibited*'."

MISCELLANEOUS

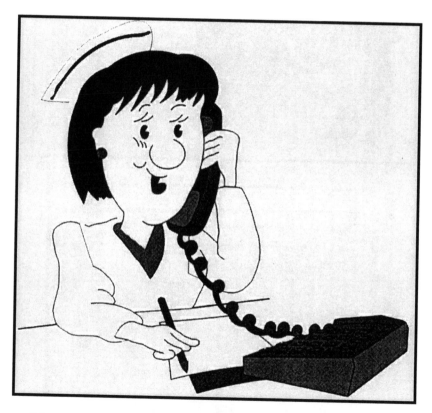

"Just wanted to confirm the order is yours, Dr. Wynn.
We've never been able to read your handwriting before.

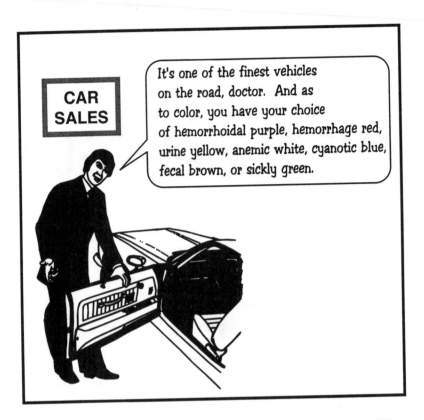

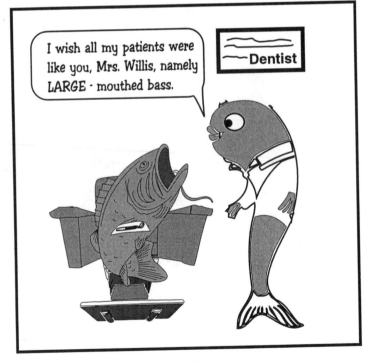

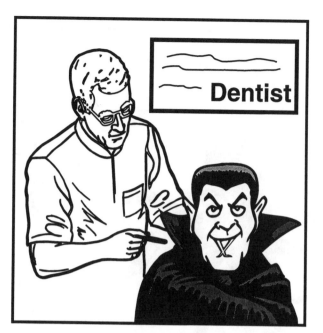

"... and you say your bite feels a little bit off?"

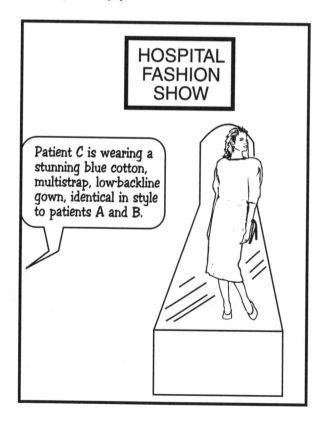

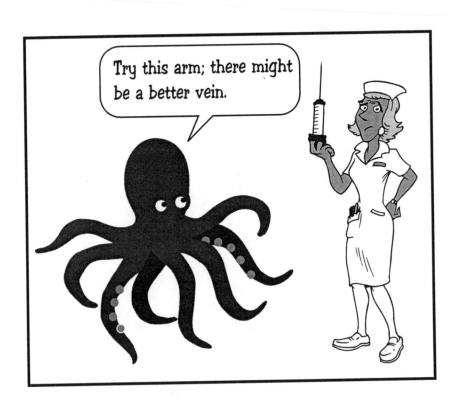

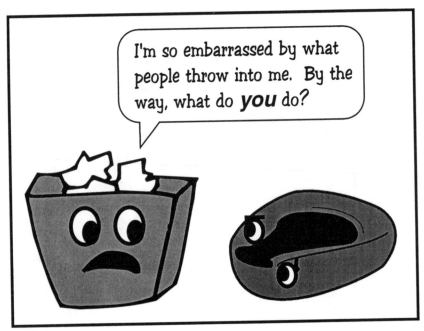

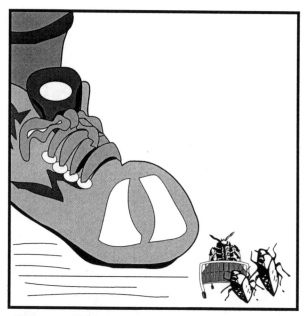

"What a filthy hospital. There are people everywhere."

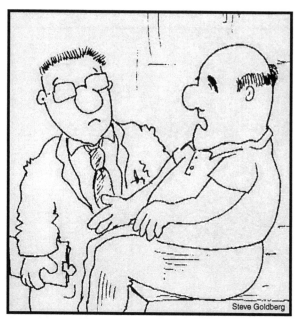

"I woke up at 3 a.m. and suddenly experienced a thrombosis of my left internal carotid artery. Tell me, Doctor, what are my symptoms?"

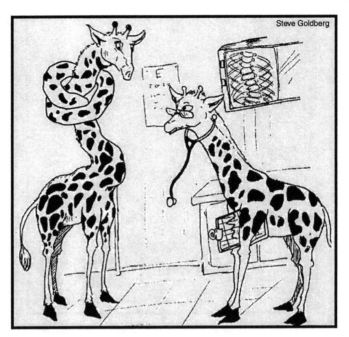

"Worst case of scoloisis I've ever seen."

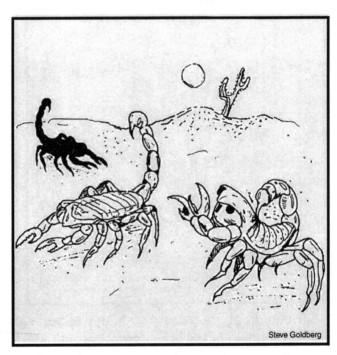

Lumbar lordosis - major killer of the desrt scorpion.

144

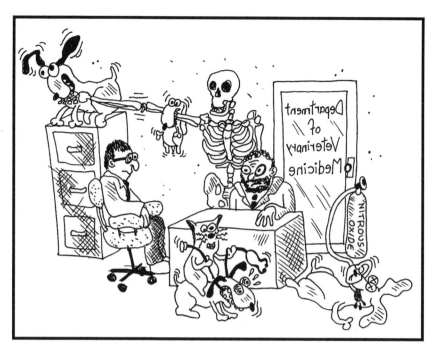

"It's been nothing but chaos since the government outlawed patient restraints."

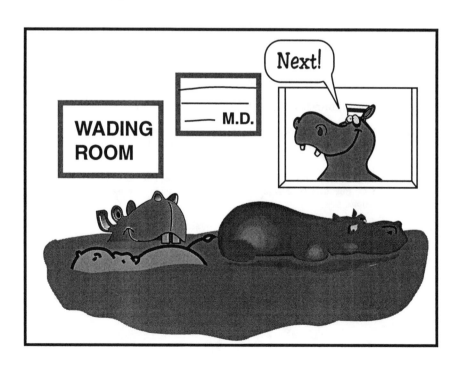